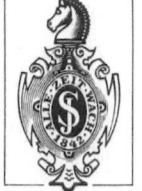

G. Jakse C. Bouffioux
J. de Leval R. A. Janknegt (Eds.)

Benign Prostatic Hyperplasia

Conservative and Operative Management

With 74 Figures and 31 Tables

Springer-Verlag Berlin Heidelberg GmbH

Prof. Dr. Gerhard Jakse

Urologische Klinik, Medizinische Fakultät der RWTH Aachen
Pauwelsstraße 30, W-5100 Aachen, FRG

Prof. Dr. Christian Bouffioux

Centre Hospitalier Universitaire, Service d'Urologie
Domaine Universitaire du Sart Tilman B 35, B-4000 Liège 1,
Belgium

Prof. Dr. Jean de Leval

Centre Hospitalier Universitaire, Service d'Urologie
Domaine Universitaire du Sart Tilman B 35, B-4000 Liège 1,
Belgium

Prof. Dr. Rudi A. Janknegt

Academisch Ziekenhuis Maastricht, Department of Urology
P. Debyelaan 25, 6202 AZ Maastricht, The Netherlands

ISBN 978-3-642-77482-9   ISBN 978-3-642-77480-5 (eBook)
DOI 10.1007/978-3-642-77480-5

Library of Congress Cataloging-in-Publication Data
Benign prostatic hyperplasia : conservative and operative management /
G. Jakse ... [et al.] (eds.). Includes bibliographical references and index.

1. Prostate—Hypertrophy. I. Jakse, G. (Gerhard) [DNLM: 1. Prostatic
Hypertrophy—therapy—congresses. WJ 752 B4672] RC899.B384 1992
616.6'506—dc20 DNLM/DLC for Library of Congress

© Springer-Verlag Berlin Heidelberg 1992
Softcover reprint of the hardcover first edition 1992

The use of general descriptive names, registered names, trademarks, etc. in this publication
does not imply, even in the absence of a specific statement, that such names are exempt from
the relevant protective laws and regulations and therefore free for general use.

Product liability: The publishers cannot guarantee the accuracy of any information about
dosage and application contained in this book. In every individual case the user must check
such information by consulting the relevant literature.

Typesetting: Storch GmbH, Wiesentheid, FRG

21/3130 – 5 4 3 2 1 0 – Printed on acid-free paper

Preface

An intense discussion has recently begun regarding current standards in the diagnosis and treatment of benign prostatic hyperplasia (BPH). A number of factors have led to this discussion.

In an increasing proportion of aging men, for example, BPH causes so-called obstructive symptoms that must be relieved by medical or operative means. This entails an immense social and economic impact in terms of health costs. In addition, recent data indicate the most frequently performed operation for BPH − transurethral resection of the prostate − is associated with a higher risk of death due to cardiac disease than open prostatectomy. Furthermore, studies using the recently developed technique of urodynamics to assess bladder outflow obstruction reveal that about 20%−30% of patients treated with transurethral resection or open prostatectomy are actually not obstructed. This means that these patients do not receive the most effective therapy. Finally, various new treatment modalities have been developed, including medical treatment directed at endocrine pathways in the prostatic cells, balloon dilatation, spirals, temporary or permanent stents, and the application of heat in hyperthermia or thermotherapy.

The contributions to this volume were selected from a symposium on the diagnosis and treatment of BPH. They are intended to provide a comprehensive review of the state of the art in treating BPH.

Aachen, Liège, Maastricht, September 1992   *The Editors*

Contents

Nonoperative Treatment

Medical Treatment

List of Contributors*

Altwein, J. E.   1, 35[1]
Bauer, H. W.   186
Baur, H.   1, 35
Bonnet, P.   178
Borchers, H.   56
Bosshardt, R.   85
Bouffioux, C.   178
Bringeon, G.   143
Cathaud, M.   143
Chapple, C. R.   95, 155
Colombo, T.   31
Dahms, S.   85
De Geeter, P.   119
Denis, L. J.   134
Devonec, M.   143
Dujardin, T.   143
Faul, P.   43
Fendler, J. P.   143
Habib, F. K.   172
Harzmann, R.   127

Heinen, G.   66
Holtermann, W.   119
Hubmer, G.   31
Jakse, G.   56, 66, 75, 85
Janknegt, R. A.   189
Kirby, R. S.   109
Laduc, R.   196
Langen, P.-H.   75
Melchior, H.-J.   119
Nordmeyer, N.   66
Perrin, P.   143
Rauchenwald, M.   31
Schäfer, W.   14, 75
Sikora, R.   85
Sohn, M.   66, 85
Vale, J. A.   109
Van Erps, P.   134
Vogt, C.   66
Weckermann, D.   127

---

* Addresses are given at the beginning of the respective contribution
[1] Page on which contribution begins

Development
of Benign Prostatic Hyperplasia

J. E. Altwein and H. Baur[1]

The prostate undergoes minimal changes until puberty. At that time, androgen stimulates the prostate to enlarge and the urethra to elongate. The prostate reaches its full size by about the age of 20 years. In the mature prostate, a marrow transition zone separates the cranial and caudal regions of the gland, and a layer of trigonal muscle descends down the front of the prostate to the verumontanum [19]. Between the ages of 20 and 40 years, the size of the prostate remains stable (Fig. 1).

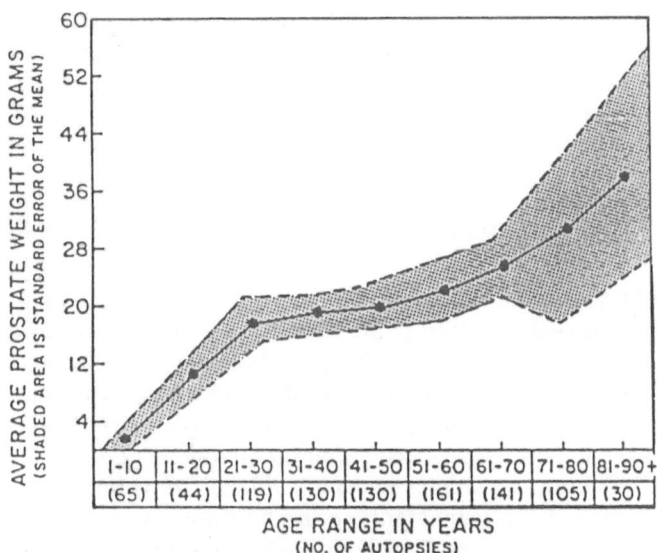

Fig. 1. Mean weight of the prostate in men of different ages. Shaded area indicates standard error of the mean for the number of glands shown. (From [3])

[1] Krankenhaus der Barmherzigen Brüder, Urologische Abteilung, Romanstraße 93, W-8000 München 19, FRG

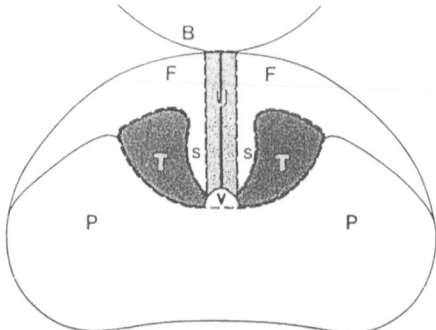

Fig. 2. Oblique coronal section of the prostate, showing the relationship between the transition zone *(T)*, periurethral region *(U)*, sphincter *(S)*, glandular prostate *(P)*, verumontanum *(V)*, anterior fibromuscular stroma *(F)*, bladder *(B)*, and urethra *(solid heavy line)*. Stippled area, the regions where BPH develops. (From [19])

After the age of 40, tiny nodules that resemble fetal mesenchyma may appear in the inner cranial zone of the prostate. The nodules coalesce and progressively constrict the caudal outer zone into a narrow rim (Fig. 2). The anatomical limits of the symphysis pubis and the bladder neck mold the swellung prostate in the classic lobes, which are pathological artifacts. In old age, carcinoma may appear in the caudal peripheral zone, outside the region where nodules of benign prostatic hyperplasia (BPH) have formed.

Etiology of BPH

Although the causes of BPH are not fully understood,it is well established that two factors are essential for the disease to develop: aging and the presence of androgenic hormones produced by functioning testes. The disease seldom occurs in men under the age of 40; nor does it occur in men who are castrated prior to puberty, and established disease sometimes regresses after orchiectomie [29].

Laboratory studies provide evidence for a hormonal basis of BPH (Tables 1, 2). Repeatedly serum hormones have been studied in BPH patients; however, problems arise when these levels are correlated to BPH, since most studies include hospilized patients, do not use morning blood sampling to account for the circadian testosterone rhythm, lack appropriate controls, and above all are not performed as case-control studies. In dogs hyperplasia can be induced by treatment with 3-alpha-androstanediol [27]. Thus research into the etiology of BPH has focused on the role of endocrine factors in controlling prostate growth.

Table 1. Correlation of age with serum hormonal factors: a survey

Decrease	Significant	Increase	Significant	Unchanged
Free testosterone	+	Sex hormone binding globulin	+	Estrogens
Androstenedione	+	Luteining hormone	+	Dihydrotestosterone
Dehydroepiandrosterone, dehydroeplandrosterone sulfate	+	Follicle-stimulating hormone	+	Testosterone
Androstenediol	+	Estrogens	−	
17-OH Pregnenolone	+			

Table 2. Correlation of BPH volume with hormonal factors (64 men subjected to radical prostatectomy)

Positive	Significant	Negative	Significant	No
Estriol	+	Androstenedione	+	Testosterone
Free Testosterone[a]	+	Corticosteroid-binding globulin[a]	+	Dihydrotestosterone
Estradiol[a]	+		+	Estrone
			−	Prolactin
				Luteinizing hormone
				Follicle-stimulating hormone
				Sex hormone binding globulin

From Partin J et al. (1991) J Urol 145:405;
[a]1 Age corrected.

A number of hypotheses have been proposed to explain the development of BPH, which are only in part linked to the action of hormones.

Risk factors for the development of BPH except aging have been investigated. So far, is no conclusive evidence as to one or the other factor being of importance, such as sexual risk factors (Table 3).

The Dihydrotestosterone Hypothesis

5-Dihydrotestosterone (DHT; Fig. 3a) has been shown to be the principal androgen controlling prostatic growth [6]. DHT is formed from testtosterone in the prostate by the enzyme 5-alpha-reductasem which is located mainly in the nuclear membrane [14]. DHT binds to androgen receptor-steroid complex, which in turn binds to DNA, inducing the synthesis of specific proteins (Fig. 4).

Table 3. Japanese-Dutch case-control study of prostatic cancer: sexual risk factors

	Results of questionnaire	Relative risk	Significantly different from	
			Hospital controls	BPH controls
reduced risk	Reduce risk More than four sexual partners before marriage fewer episodes of sexually transmitted diseases	0.35 0.36	+	+
increased risk	Increased risk Coitus more than five per week third decade fourth decade less frequent orgasm	2.89 2.26 2.55 4.96	+ + +	+

From Dishi et al. (1990)

In most species the ability of the prostate to synthesize DHT declines with age; the only exceptions are those species which develop benign hyperplasia. The concentration of DHT in human prostate glands showing hyperplasia has been reported to be significantly higher than that in normal glands, with higher concentrations in hyperplastic regions of diseased glands than in normal regions [23]. These findings led to the suggestion that the development of BPH was linked to an accumulation of DHT in the prostate [23]. Subsequent work showed that administration of a DHT precursor, 3-alpha-androstanediol to dogs led to prostatic hyperplasia, with the same pathological features as those occurring spontaneously in aging animals [11, 27].

The putative role of DHT in the pathogenesis of BPH has recently been questioned: Walsh et al. [28] measured DHT concentrations in normal and hyperplastic tissues obtained during surgery and found that there was no significant difference in the DHT concentration in the two types of tissue. Moreover, concentrations of DHT in tissues obtained at autopsy − the source of tissue used in previous studies − were lower than those in freshly obtained tissue. This suggests that DHT is unlikely to have a major causative role in the development of BPH, although several lines of evidence favor a permissive role. Most studies of prostatic steroid metabolism indicate that there is a shift toward DHT formation in hyperplastic tissue compared with normal tissue [22]. There is

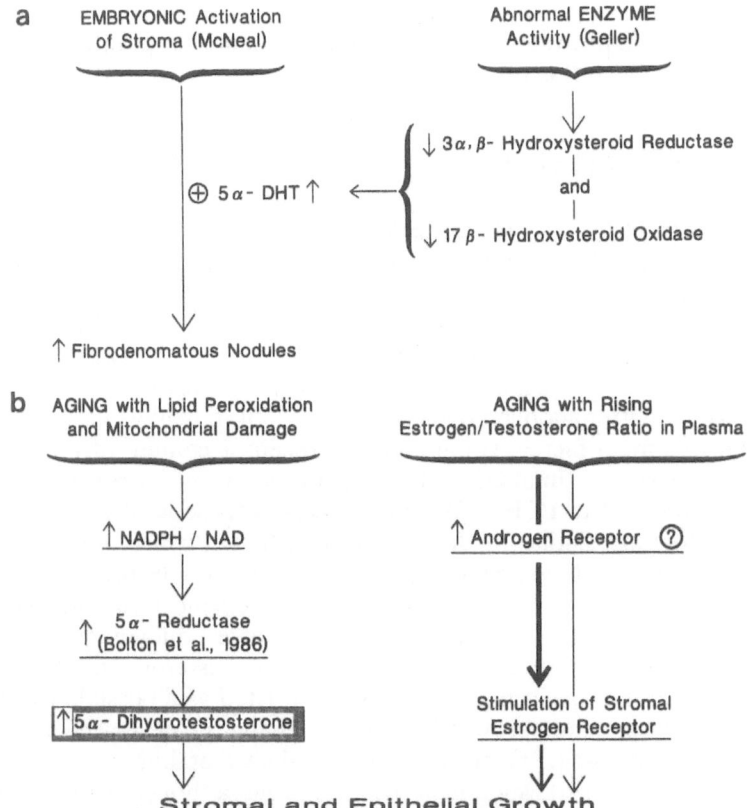

Fig. 3a, b. Hypothetic pathogenesis of BPH. **a** Dihydrotestosterone hypothesis.
b Estrogen hypothesis

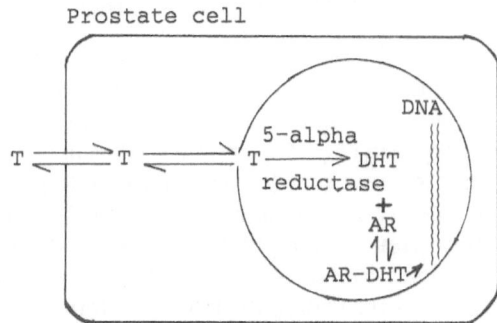

Fig. 4. Formation of dihydrotestosterone *(DHT)* from testosterone *(T)* in the prostate, binding of DHT to the androgen receptor *(AR)*, and interaction of the DHT
receptor complex with DNA

also evidence in dogs for a change in the responsiveness of the hyperplastic prostate to DHT, leading to enhanced proliferation and decreased secretion [23].

The Estrogen Hypothesis

Estrogens (Fig. 3b) are considered to have a synergistic role with androgens in the control of prostate growth and thus are potential candidates for involvement in the development of BPH. In dogs, concurrent treatment with estradiol and androstandediol causes hyperplasia, although estradiol alone has no effect [11, 27]. Furthermore, hyperplasia is more marked after treatment with estrogens and androgens than after andogen treatment alone [30], possibly because estrogen treatment increases the andogen receptor content of the canine prostate [17]. In humans, prostatic androgen receptor concentrations are increased in BPH [25], but the concentrations of progesterone receptors are similar to those in normal tissue, which indicates that estrogens do not have a direct stimulatory effect on the prostate. There is a slight decrease in circulating testosterone concentrations in aging men, which is not accompanied by a corresponding decrease in estradiol concentrations. Thus the ratio of testosterone to estradiol is changed, and this change has often been cited as a possible cause of abnormal prostatic growth [13]. These changes can, however, occur after the onset of BPH, and hence it is unlikely that they are responsible for initiating the development of hyperplasia, although they may help to maintain the hyperplastic process.

The Embryonic Reawaking Hypothesis

Evidence suggests that the responsiveness of the prostate to androgens might depend on the ratio of epithelial cells to stromal cells within the gland, both during normal development and the development of hyperplasia (Fig. 4). Animal studies have shown that, although androgens are necessary for normal prostate growth, they are not sufficient per se. In adult rodents, for example, the prostate does not continue to grow after reaching maturity despite the presence of high circulating concentrations of male sex hormones, and exogenous androgens do not cause overgrowth of the adult prostate [10]. In the embryo, the glandular portion of the prostate is derived from prostatic buds, which arise from the urethra and invade the embryonic stroma (= mesenchyma). Eventually, the mesenchyma becomes filled with epithelial tissue and

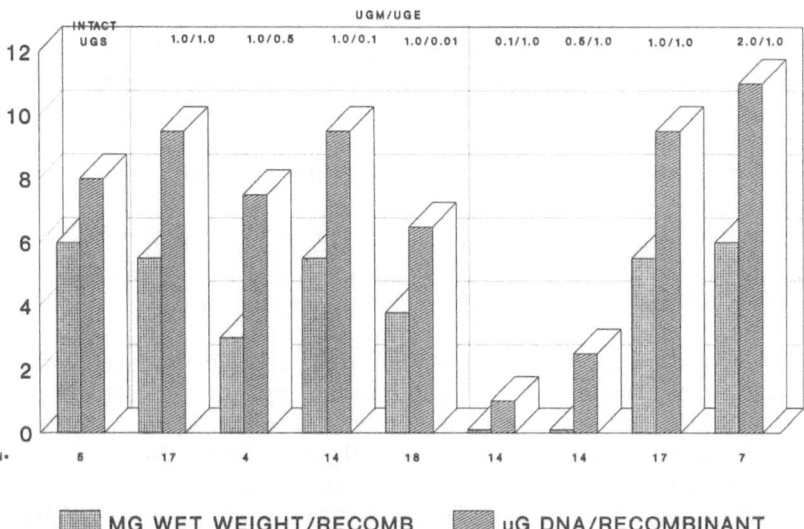

Fig. 5. Urogenital sinus mesenchyma induction of prostate growth: weight dependance. (From [9])

growth stops, which suggests that the final size of the gland is determined by the amount of stromal tissue initially present.

Experimental studies have shown that the androgens act on the stroma to induce epithelial growth, rather than directly on the epithelium. In rat prostate, glandular growth from small ductal fragments has been shown to occur only when the fragments are grafted with urogenital mesenchyma (Fig. 5; [8]). This induction of epithelial growth by stroma depends on the presence of androgens.

Evidence for the role of epithelial-stromal interactions in the development of BPH is provided by the morphological studies of McNeal [20]. These studies show that the initial change in BPH involves the formation of glandular nodules, which branch and invade the stroma in a similar manner to that seen in the embryonic gland. McNeal has suggested that the ability of stromal tissue to induce epithelial growth might be „reawakened" during adulthood in men who eventually develop BPH. Subsequent investigators have shown that the amount of stromal tissue is increased in BPH [21].

Effects of Growth Factors. The interactions between different cell types in the prostate may involve diffusible growth factors. A number of growth factors have been identified in normal and hyperplastic prostatic tissue, including epidermal growth factor (EGF) and fibroblast growth factor [13]. Prostate cells in culture proliferate in response to EGF, transforming growth factors, and other peptides, such as insulin and prolactin. There is an inverse relationship between androgen receptors and EGF receptors in normal and hyperplastic tissue, and hyperplasia is associated with changes in the proportion of high- and low-affinity EGF receptors [13].

The Stem-Cell Hypothesis

The stem-cell hypothesis suggests that BPH arises from an imbalance between the growth of new cells and the maturation and death of older cells [15]. In the normal prostate, the rates of cell proliferation and cell death are in equilibrium. The stem cells divide to produce a pool of actively proliferating cells, which mature into functional, non-proliferating cells and eventually die. BPH might develop as a result of either an increase in the number of stem cells or a failure of the pro-liferating cells to mature and die. These defects might be „imprinted" in the stem cells during critical periods of development.

Natural History

BPH is most common in men over 50 years of age, elthough studies of prostates obtained at autopsy or on prostatectomy indicates that the hyperplastic process may begin before the age of 30 [3], with a phase of accelerated growth at about 40 years of age. Growth then continues throughout life, although it is not known whether any hyperplastic glands show spontaneous regression [4]. About 50% of men have BPH by the age of 60 years, and by the age of 90 the incidence may be as high as 90%. Although the first pathological signs can be seen in autopsy specimens from men aged 31–40 years, the incidence is low in this age group (8%).

The age-related changes in prostate size have been studied by Berry et al. [3], who analyzed the data from ten studies in which prostates were obtained at autopsy or during prostatectomy. These authors iden-tified two phases of prostatic growth: an initial spurt during puberty and maturation, followed by a period of slower growth throughout later life (Fig. 1). The mean weight of normal adult prostates in this study was 20 g; this weight increased to 33 g in glands with PBH. Large prostates, however, were relatively uncommon; only 4% of prostates in men aged 70 years or over weighed more than 100 g. Regression analysis revealed that the theoretical doubling time for BPH was 4.5 years in men aged between 31 and 50 years and over 100 years in men aged over 70.

Morphological Development

McNeal [20] studied the morphological development of BPH and found that is was confined to the periurethral and transition zones, proximal to the verumontanum and close to the cylindrical urinary sphincter (Fig. 2). The earliest pathological sign of BPH is the occurrence os small, spherical nodules, which arise in the transition zone and are composed ob both glandular and stromal tissue. Growth of these nodules and diffuse enlargement of the transition zone follows as the disease progresses [20]. Periurethral nodules tend to be smaller and are usually derived from the stroma. The formation of hyperplastic nodules usually begins with proliferation of fibroplasts, to form clusters. These clusters are subsequently invaded by other cell types, such as glandular epithelial cells, smooth muscle cells, and myoepithelial cells, resulting in discruption of the normal relationship between these cells [30]. As the disease progresses, large nodules replace the normal prostatic tissue, which is reduced to a thin peripheral rim. Small cells and areas of infarction can sometimes be found within the nodules [26].

Histological changes occur in all components of the prostate during development of BPH. The proportion of secretory columnar cells within each glandular acinus is decreased, and the proportion of fibroblasts is increased. The stroma of hyperplastic glands does not possess the elastic tissue found in the normal gland. Secondary changes can occur as a result of BPH [26]. These include cystic dilatation of the acini and ducts, accompanied by atrophy of the epithelium and lymphoid infiltration of the stroma.

The observation that BPH develops only within a small, localized area of the prostate might provide clues to the pathogenesis of the disease. It has been shown that BPH originates in the periurethral glandular tissue at the verumontanum, the point where the ejaculatory ducts enter the urethra, and suggests that glands in this region are derived from the wolffian duct, whereas glandular tissue elsewhere in the prostate is derived from the urogenital sinus [4, 18, 19]. This would suggest that, in humans at least, BPH develops in a unique population of cells [30].

Development of Symptoms

The clinical symptoms of BPH result from obstruction of the urethra by an enlarged prostate. Although autopsy studies show that pathological signs of BPH are common in elderly men, only 10% – 25% of those with pathological signs of the disease develop symptoms that require surgery [4, 16]. This is a consequence of the periurethral origin of BPH. In the early stages of the disease, hyperplasia is not always symmetrical about the urethra. Compression of the urethra by hyperplastic tissue can give rise to obstruction before the hyperplasia has extended beyond the prostatic capsule. As the disease progresses, the hyperplastic tissue can expand both inwards, compressing the urethra, and outwards, compressing the true glandular tissue against the capsule. In advanced disease, the true glandular tissue is replaced by hyperplastic tissue, and the urethra is significantly narrowed, producing increasingly severe symptoms. Conversely, obstruction of the urethra can occur as a result of regional changes within the prostate, in the absence of an overall change in size [24]. Thus there is only a poor correlation between the presence of symptoms and the size of the prostate [8].

Urinary obstruction in BPH has two components [7]: a relatively constant mechanical component, resulting from physical compression of the urethra, and a dynamic component, which depends on the tone of the prostatic smooth muscle.

Estimates of the number of men requiring surgery for symptomatic relief vary. Birkhoff concluded that a 50-year-old man has a 20% – 25% chance of undergoing a prostatectomy during his lifetime [4]. These estimates are consistent with the findings of the Veterans Administration Normative Aging Study, which concluded that the lifetime probability of undergoing surgery for BPH is 29% [12].

A number of studies have examined the clinical course of untreated BPH [2, 5]. Most have shown considerable variation in the severity of symptoms as the disease progresses. Birkhoff et al. [5] followed a group of 26 patients prospectively for 3 years. In this study, 15 patients reported that their symptoms deteriorated, and 8 reported improvement; when measured objectively, however, symptoms were seen to deteriorate in 20 patients and improve in only 4 patients. Moreover, deterioration was slow and fluctuating. Symptoms of BPH generally worsen, although temporary improvement is occasionally seen. In another study, involving 97 patients, symptoms were unchanged or improved over 5 years in 84%, and only 10% showed disease progression that was sufficiently severe to warrant surgery. The most informative data were recently reported by Arrighi et al. [1] from the Baltimore Longitudinal Study of Aging (Fig. 6).

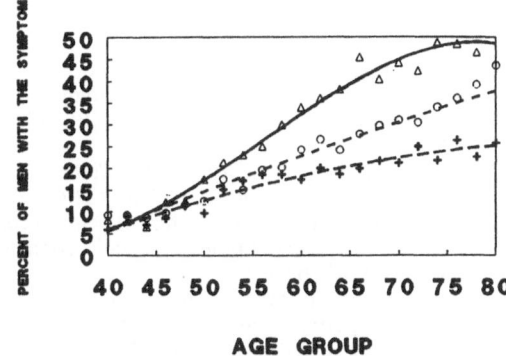

Fig. 6. Data from the Baltimore Longitudinal Study of Aging. (From [1])
△—△, change in size/farce, ○—○ incomplete emplying, +—+ hesilancy

Conclusion

BPH is most common in men aged over 50 years, although the hyperplastic process may be initiated before the age of 30. The first pathological change in BPH is the formation of nodules of hyperplastic tissue in the transitional and periurethral zones of the prostate. In advanced disease, these nodules can replace the normal prostatic tissue. There is little correlation between the degree of hyperplasia and the severity of symptoms. BPH is a progressive disease, although there is evidence that remissions can occur. If untreated, a number of sequelae and complications may develop, including detrusor decompensation, urinary tract infections, and hydronephrosis.

The etiology of BPH is not fully understood. Research has focused on the role of hormones, particularly androgens, in controlling the growth of the prostate. The DHT hypothesis suggests that accumulation of DHT within the prostate is associated with the development of BPH. Although DHT may not be a direct pathogenic factor, it is likely to play a permissive role. Similarly, a change in the ratio of estrogens to androgens may contribute to the maintenance of hyperplasia. Another view is that hyperplasia might result from an increased ability of stromal tissue to induce epithelial growth, and that prostatic growth factors might also be involved in the development of BPH. The stem-cell hypothesis suggests that BPH results from an imbalance between the rates of cell proliferation and cell maturation and death.

References

1. Arrighi HM, Guess HA, Metter EJ, Fozard JL (1990) Symptoms and signs of prostatism as risk factors for prostatectomy. Prostate 16:253−261
2. Ball AJ, Feneley RCL, Abrams PH (1981) The natural history of untreated ‚prostatism'. Br J Urol 53:613−616
3. Berry SJ, Coffey DS, Walsh PC et al. (1984) The development of human benign prostatic hyperplasia with age. J Urol 132:474−479
4. Birkhoff JD (1983) Natural history of benign prostatic hypertrophy. In: Hinman F Jr, Boyarsky S (eds) Benign prostatic hypertrophy. Springer, Berlin Heidelberg New York, pp 5−9
5. Birkhoff JD, Wiederkorn AR, Hamilton ML (1976) Natural history of benign prostatic hypertrophy and acute urinary retention. Urology 7:48−52
6. Bruchowsky N, Wilson JD (1968) The conversion of testosterone to 5α-androstan-17β-ol-3-one by rat prostate in vivo and in vitro. J Biol Chem 243:2012−2021
7. Caine M (1986) The present role of alpha-adrenergic blockers in the treatment of benign prostatic hypertrophy. J Urol 136:1−4
8. Chapman L, Lapi N, Fethiere W (1964) Prostatic enlargement and lower urinary tract obstruction. Geriatrics 19:231
9. Chung LWK, Cuner GR (1983) Stromal-epithelial interactions: II. Regulation of prostatic growth by embryonic urogenital sinus mesenchyme. Prostate 4:503−511
10. Cunha GR et al. (1987) The endocrinology and developmental biology of the prostate. Endocr Rev 8:338−362
11. deKlerk DP, Coffey DS, Ewing LL et al. (1979) Comparison of spontaneous and experimentally induced canine prostatic hyperplasia. J Clin Invest 64:842−849
12. Glynn RJ, Campion EW, Bouchard GR et al. (1985) The development of benign prostatic hyperplasia among volunteers in the Normative Aging Study. Am J Epidemiol 121:78−90
13. Griffiths K, Davies P, Eaton C et al. (1991) Endocrine factors in the initiation, diagnosis and treatment of prostatic cancer. In: Voight KD, Knabbe C (eds) Endocrine dependent tumors. Raven, New York, 83−130
14. Houston B, Chisholm GD, Habib FK (1985) Evidence that human prostatic 5α-reductase is located exclusively in the nucleus. FEBS Lett 1985:231−235
15. Isaacs JT, Coffey DS (1989) Etiology and disease process of benign prostatic hyperplasia. Prostate 2 [Suppl]:33−50
16. Lytton B, Emery JM, Harvard BM (1968) The incidence of benign prostatic obstruction. J Urol 99:639−645
17. Moore RJ, Gazak JM, Wilson JD (1979) Regulation of cytoplasmic dihydrotestosterone binding in dog prostate by 17B-β-estradiol. J Clin Invest 63:351
18. McNeal JE (1972) The prostate and prostatic urethra: a morphologic synthesis. J Urol 107:1008−1016
19. McNeal JE (1975) Development and comparative anatomy of the prostate. In: Grayhack JT, Wilson JD, Sherbenske MJ (eds) Benign prostatic hyperplasia. DHEW publication no (NIH) 76−1113, Washington, pp 1−9
20. McNeal JE (1978) Origin and evolution of benign prostatic enlargement. Invest Urol 15:340−345
21. Rohr HP, Bartsch G (1980) Human benign prostatic hyperplasia: a stromal disease? Urology 16:625
22. Romijn JC (1989) Steroid hormones, receptors, and benign prostatic hyperplasia. New Dev Biosci 5:63−72

23. Siiteri PK, Wilson JD (1970) Dihydrotestosterone in prostatic hypertrophy: I. The information and content dihydrotestosterone in the hypertrophic prostate of man. J Clin Invest 49:1737–1745
24. Turner Warwick R et al. (1973) A urodynamic view of prostatic obstruction and the results of prostatectomy. Br J Urol 45:631–645
25. van Aubel OGJM, Bolt-de Vries J, Blankenstein MA et al. (1985) Nuclear androgen receptor content in biopsy speciments from histologically normal, hyperplastic and cancerous human prostate tissue. Prostate 6:185–194
26. Varma V et al. (1989) Prostate and seminal vesicles. In: Someren A (ed) Urologic pathology with clinical and radiologic correlations. Macmillan, New York, pp 467–533
27. Walsh PC, Wilson JD (1976) The induction of prostatic hypertrophy in the dog with androstanediol. J Clin Invest 57:1093–1097
28. Walsh PC, Hutchins GM, Ewing LL (1983) Tissue content of dihydrotestosterone in human prostatic hyperplasia is not supranormal. J Clin Invest 72:1772·1777
29. Walsh PC et al. (1987) Steroid receptors and dihydrotestosterone content in human normal and benign hyperplastic prostatic tissue. In: Rodgers CH et al. (eds) Benign prostatic hyperplasia, vol II. NIH publication no 87-2881, Washington, pp 153–159
30. Wilson JD (1980) The pathogenesis of benign prostatic hyperplasia. Am J Med 68:745–756

Bladder Outflow Obstruction: Definition, Clinical Application, and Grading in Benign Prostatic Hyperplasia

W. Schäfer[1]

Introduction

A discussion about „obstruction" in urology is hampered by rather vague and unspecific terminology. The term „obstruction" itself is used in many different ways and meanings for the upper and lower urinary tract. There seems to exist agreement that obstruction denotes a change in function to inefficient function with potential damage of the lower tract and danger for the upper tract. The same term „obstruction" is also used for accompanying symptoms and morphological alterations presumably causing and/or caused by obstruction.

In this way obstruction may refer to: *obstructive symptoms* of benign prostatic hyperplasia (BPH), such as a weak stream, hesitancy, interrupted voiding, straining, postvoiding dribbling, feeling of incomplete emptying with residual urine volume; *obstructive morphology* such as the finding of an enlarged prostate either by rectal digital examination, some imaging procedure, or endoscopy, where even different forms and degrees of obstruction are sometimes described. Obstruction may refer to *indicators of obstruction* such as postvoiding residual volume, bladder trabeculation, the range of irritative bladder symptoms and nocturia, or its effects on the upper tract, with reflux and dilatation [8].

Since objective measurement of bladder voiding function has become established, it is possible to define normal and to identify abnormal function. All sound studies, using slightly different concepts of obstruction, show major disagreement between these presumably specific symptoms, morphological findings and other indicators of obstruction, and the result from urodynamic measurement and data analysis [3, 4, 9, 22, 23, 28]. A common conclusion from this disagreement is that the value of urodynamics is limited, and that the urodynamic definition of obstruction is unrealistic or clinically irrelevant, or even that in BPH it actually does not matter because the

[1] Urologische Klinik, Medizinische Fakultät der RWTH, Pauwelsstraße 30, W-5100 Aachen, FRG

symptoms alone justify surgery. I think the proper conclusion is that the only scientifically acceptable and sound approach is an objective definition of obstruction based on measurable parameters alone because of the limited reliability and specificity of the traditional „confirmations" of obstruction [23, 24, 28]. Such an objective definition of obstruction must start with a clear concept of normal voiding function, a clear description of the contributing parameters and how they can be measured, and then lead to a concept for data interpretation, first on a physical level, then on a patho-physiological level, and only then on a clinical level [14].

Normal Voiding Function

Normal voiding is achieved by detrusor contraction initiated at sphincter relaxation, which means that the active component is the detrusor, and the outlet is passive. In a combination of an active and passive component is meaningful to assume that the active component has at least a major contribution to voiding function. Therefore, I concentrate first on the discussion of active detrusor function.

In urodynamics the muscular activity of the detrusor is measured as pressure and flow rate, and it is rather easy to calculate the original muscular parameters of force and contraction velocity from the urodynamic values [2, 11, 17, 18]. The important point is that the muscle does not separately generate a force or a velocity but both together as mechanical muscle power (P), which according to the specific working conditions for the muscle is converted to pressure (p) and flow rate (Q). This can be described formally as: $P = p \times Q$.

This simple equation says that for a given detrusor power (P) a high flow rate (Q) is possible only at a low pressure (p), and that a low flow rate occurs at a high pressure. If a low flow rate occurs at a low pressure, it is obvious that this must be due to a low detrusor power (Fig. 1).

Voiding means for the detrusor to do work. It can be shown that the amount of energy available for the detrusor to do work in one contraction cycle is limited [11]. Power is work per unit of time. It the power is spent with high pressure and low flow rate, only a small volume is voided after a period of time, i.e., with the same work which normally yields a large volume. Normal, i.e., ideal voiding can be discussed in terms of voiding efficiency (Eff) of the lower urinary tract, defined as the volume voided related to the amount of work needed to transport the volume through the outlet [13], or in dynamic terms as the flow rate (Q) achieved by a certain muscle power (P). This can be very simply written as:

$$\text{Eff} = \frac{Q}{P} = \frac{Q}{p \times Q} = \frac{1}{p}$$

This makes clear on a simple physical/biomechanical level that the conceptualization of efficient voiding function is characterized by the voiding detrusor pressure, and that efficiency is inversely related to the detrusor pressure, i.e., a high efficiency means a low pressure and vice versa. I think it important for the reevaluation of traditional urological thinking to realize that not flow rate but pressure is the key parameter to define obstruction.

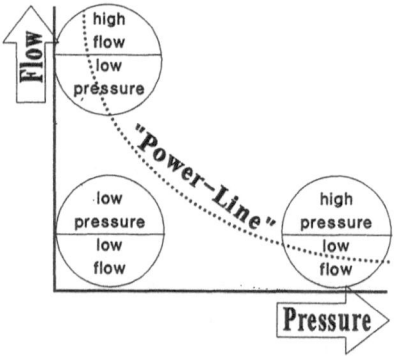

Fig. 1. In a graph of pressure versus flow rate a line of the same mechanical power *(power line)* is a hyperbola. Such a graphical presentation of the equation
$P = p \times Q$ constant
is a simple first approximation, as it is clear that for the extreme values of maximum pressure and maximum flow rate physiological limits do apply while the equation would yield infinitesimely high values. The graph shows clearly the inverse relation of pressure and flow rate for a given power as well as the result of a very weak detrusor with low power

Obstruction

The quality of voiding can be judged immediately by flow rate recording alone, but the cause of a poor voiding cannot be itentified from the flow rate alone. A weak detrusor voids very efficiently through a normal outlet with a low flow rate at a low pressure. But the same low flow rate can be achieved from a normal detrusor through an obstructed outlet at high pressure. Therefore I have introduced „voiding efficiency" as the flow-related muscle power required to transport urine through the outlet, so that we can define „obstructed" as „inefficient" voiding function, with the cause of this increased demand for voiding power clearly located in the bladder outlet [13].

Effects of Obstruction

The elevated voiding pressure at obstruction has traditionally been interpreted as a sign of „compensatory hypertrophy" of the detrusor, meaning that the detrusor becomes stronger, i.e., more powerful, under load. Without discussing the complex histomorphological changes seen in the detrusor under obstruction, the introduction of mechanical voiding power allows a simple but realistic judgement about a change in detrusor function. The result is clear: elevated pressure is the consequence of the change in working conditions under obstruction, of the reduced flow rate for a detrusor of unchanged power [5, 10, 11]. This means that effective „compensatory detrusor hypertrophy" is not a general and typical feature of BPH, and it is not clear whether it exists at all in BPH. There is a very simple clinical confirmation of this urodynamic finding. If the muscle power would increase in reaction to BPH obstruction, normalization of outflow conditions by surgery must result in a higher than normal flow rate at normal pressure. Obviously a normal flow rate is the best possible and typical result after transurethral resection of the prostate. Another feature of obstruction is residual postvoiding urine. Our simple approach allows a clear answer: the detrusor actually does more work under obstruction, but not enough to compensate the increased demand up to complete voiding. This means that maximum potential work which the detrusor can do is not very different between obstructed and normal voiding condition. Thus, under obstruction all energy is consumed before the bladder is emptied completely so that the occurrence of residual urine is clearly due to exhaustion of the detrusor [11].

Different Forms of Obstruction

Ideal bladder outflow conditions are characterized by minimal energy requirement for urine transport, which in physical terms is a large, effective minimal cross-sectional area and a low opening pressure of the flow-controlling zone, and in physiological terms a wide and easily opening urethra. This can be depicted clearly in a pressure/flow graph and results urodynamically in a low voiding detrusor pressure at high flow rate. A smaller effective cross-sectional area and an elevated opening pressure both lead to an increased energy demand for urine outflow. The two changes do occur separately, are related to distinctly different pathological changes, and lead to different types of obstruction with different consequences for the lower urinary tract [12]. The constrictive obstruction seen with strictures affect only the effective

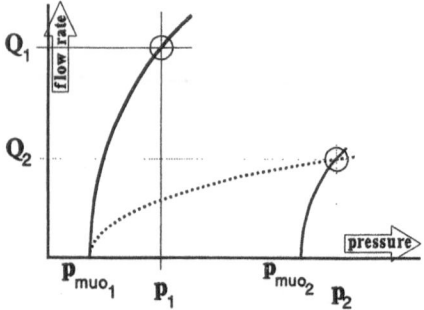

Fig. 2. Normal voiding starts at a low urethral opening pressure (p_{muo1}) and yield the maximum pressure (p_1) with the flow rate (Q_1) dependent on the detrusor power. Obstruction means a higher pressure with a lower flow rate. A constrictive obstruction has a normal opening pressure (p_{muo1}) but has a flat shape according to the reduced lumen size, so that the low peak flow (Q_2) needs a high pressure (p_2). A compressive obstruction is characterized by an elevated opening pressure (p_{muo2}), and although it may lead to the same reduced flow rate and elevated pressure as the constrictive type, it is a more severe form of obstruction because at pressures below p_{muo2} no voiding is possible. This elevated minimal pressure is the most critical parameter for development of postvoiding residual urine volumes

cross-sectional area and lead to the typical plateaulike flow rate curve. The compressive obstruction seen in BPH affect mainly the minimal urethral opening pressure and lead to the typical flattened, asymmetric flow curve with a trailing end. Although the low flow rate may occur at the same elevated obstructive voiding pressure, there is a distinct and relevant difference between these two types of obstruction toward the termination of voiding (Fig. 2).

In neurogenic obstruction with dyssynergic conditions, the sphincter can contract and lead to premature detrusor inhibition. When we exclude here neurogenic forms of obstruction, voiding is terminated either when the bladder is empty, or when the detrusor can no longer generate the minimal voiding pressure [1, 11, 13]. It is obvious that the demand for minimal voiding power is elevated in a compressive obstruction, which explains why BPH is much more likely to be accompanied by residual urine that a plain urethral stricture.

Urodynamic Data Analysis

The reliability and quality of the potential information derived from measurement are clearly limited by two factors mainly, the quality of the original data and that of the analytical procedure applied. It is obviously dangerous to use a sophisticated analysis on poor data, as it may be misleading to use an inadequate, simple method to exploit good data [7].

The quality of urodynamic data which can be realistically collected under clinical circumstances is far from ideal, and we must use an analytical model which takes account of such limitations. Minimal psychological interference, repeated measurement to exclude artifacts and assess intraindividual variability, using slow or even natural bladder filling, and identification of „normal" voiding volume from a voiding diary or voiding at different volumes are all important steps for improving signal quality. Such refinements are relevant when minor changes are to be detected, such as those expected from drugs and when sophisticated computer analysis is planned [12, 13, 15, 25, 26]. Surgery introduces dramatic changes to voiding function, so that a more pragmatic approach to measurement and a less precise but more robust approach to data analysis is justified.

The aim of urodynamic data analysis must be the realistic qualification of the mechanical voiding balance with clearcut quantification of the contribution of the bladder outlet, irrespective of or at least not substantially dependent on detrusor contraction function. Griffiths' suggestion to plot pressure versus flow rate was an important first step to realistic interpretation of the pressure/flow relationship from the traditional urodynamic recordings of pressures and flow rate over time [1, 5, 20]. These plots have made clear how complex the pressure/flow relation of urinary voiding can be, and that the traditional „urethral resistance factors" can at best be considered a very poor, potentially misleading interpretation of the data. These p/Q plots, however, allowed only a qualitative descriptive judgement without any clear quantification. The passive urethral resistance relation (PURR) was the first adequate quantitative approach using a realistic physical and physiological model to assess the bladder outlet function [12, 13, 21]. Different from the simple single resistance factors, the PURR requires two parameters to define the „two-dimensional" balance between urethra and detrusor. Later, Spangberg et al. tried to come to an even closer approximation of the real pressure/flow relation, which yielded a three-parameter model for bladder outflow function [15, 27]. Both models, the PURR and the three-parameter model depend on computer application and are sensitive to artifacts as discussed before.

In addition, the resultant two or three parameters make possible an easy comparative classification of different voidings only when all of these parameters are different in the same way. If one parameter relates to better and the other to worse outflow conditions, a clear comparative judgement of outflow conditions is impossible. This is not an error in the models but reflects the difficulty in curve analysis when dif-

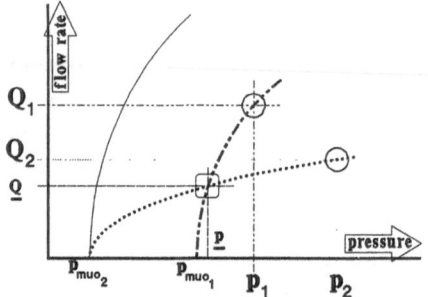

Fig. 3. Two parameters are needed to define the PURR, the opening pressure (p_{muo}) and the slope of the curve. If the curves cross, it is difficult to decide which one establishes a stronger obstruction because the resultant pressure/flow relations are superimposed. Furthermore, in such a case the degree of obstruction depends on the detrusor strength. For the range below the values p/Q, it is clear that the compressive obstruction is more severe, because all flow values occur at pressures higher than p_{muo1}. Above these values p/Q a stronger detrusor contraction yields less flow rate in the constrictive type, with Q_2 being lower than Q_1 at a pressure p_2 higher than p_1. Therefore, such different types of obstruction can be compared only for a given volume and given detrusor strength and ultimately only by calculation of the actual energy spent

ferent pressure/flow plots are not clearly separate but are crossing or superimposed.

The derived parameters quantify certain aspects of outlet mechanics, such as opening pressure, effective cross-sectional area, and elasticity, and it is obvious that different combinations of these parameters cannot be clearly related to the resultant outflow conditions. A constrictive and a compressive PURR, i.e., the combination of a low opening pressure and a small cross-sectional area and the combination of a high opening pressure and a large cross-sectional area are distinctly different outflow conditions and show a distinctly different pressure/flow pattern in the urodynamic recording. However, this does not necessarily imply that a definite classification as more or less obstructed with respect to effectively different urodynamic voiding function can be derived from this analysis (Fig. 3).

These difficulties can be largely circumvented on the basis of disease-specific forms of outflow obstruction. Typical for BPH is the compressive form of obstruction, and the characteristic aspect of compressive obstruction is the minimum urethral opening pressure (p_{muo}). Thus, when ignoring the differences in the slope of the PURR, which are of minor importance in BPH, a clear classification of prostatic obstruction becomes possible using the p_{muo} value alone [22, 23]. Similar is the concept of the group-specific resistance factor (URA; [6]), based on the observation that the slope of the PURR is related to the opening pressure, so that both parameters can be combined in a single number through statistical procedures. This URA is thus a single parameter, in essence the „statistical opening pressure", which allows clear grading but with the disadvantage that deviations from the underlying „ideal statistical" relation are obscured and can yield misleading results [16, 19].

The Pressure/Flow Diagram

From the experience that detailed analysis of voiding function is possible but does not lead reliably to the data needed for clinical decision making, further steps of simplification have been introduced with the „linear PURR" and the pressure/flow diagram [24]. The linear PURR follows the results that the curvature of the pressure/flow curve and the PURR or the three-parameter model are not very well reproducible in detail, and that these details hardly affect voiding function [15]. They may offer scientifically interesting information of outlet function, but they do not provide relevant information for clinical classification of outflow obstruction beyond the disease-specific identification of the typical compressive form of obstruction in BPH. A straight line therefore suggests itself as the simplest form of a curve and a rough approximation of the actual slope. The real advantage is that a linear pressure/flow curve can be constructed without computer use in a simple, manual, graphic procedure because construction of a straight line requires only two data points. This simple methos needs only to identify the two critical points of the linear PURR, i.e., the pressure at maximum flow and the equivalent to the original p_{muo} the lowest pressure at initiation or termination of flow. Unfortunately, this is not as simple as it appears because it is essential to make proper corrections for the time delay when flow is recorded in the flowmeter with respect to the time when pressure is measured [12]. This is particularly relevant when pressure changes rapidly. Especially at the end of voiding, when the lowest voiding pressure is commonly found, it is necessary to eliminate the last 5 ml at very low flow rate of less than 2 ml/s leaving the distal urethra after the proximal prostatic flow controlling zone is already closed [25] (Fig. 4).

Grading Outflow Function

We have designed a pressure/flow diagram which uses groups of data for grading obstruction instead of distinct single values and in this way

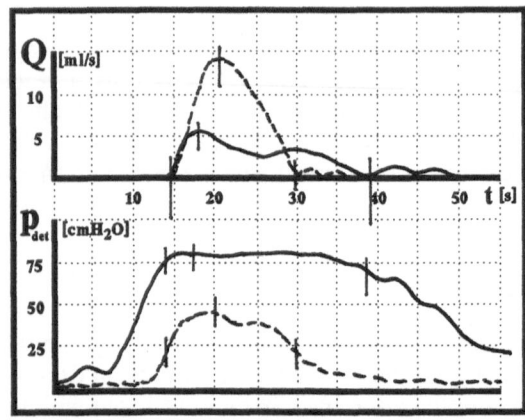

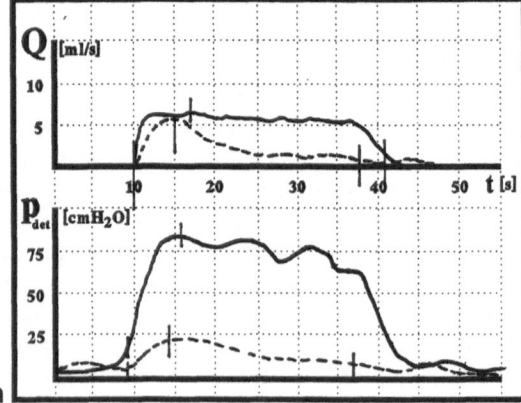

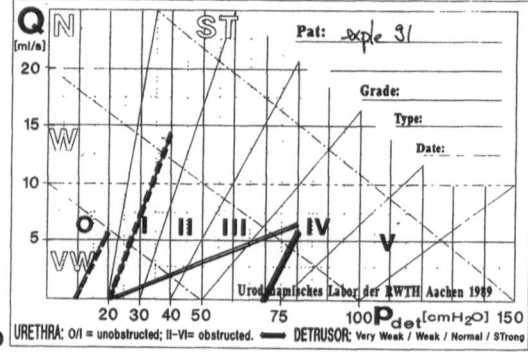

correct for the normal intraindividual variability as well as putting the linear approximation into proper perspective. This diagram takes into account the increasing slope of the PURR with higher opening pressure. Furthermore, some useful aspects of clinical applicability have been integrated (see Fig. 4).

The group 0 is rather large because all patients in this group are definitely unobstructed, and there is no need for further differentiation. Groups I−III are the most interesting both because they comprise most prostatic patients, and because they contain the critical border between obstructed and unobstructed. The width of these groups is simplified to 10 cm H_2O, which is very close to the range of intraindividual variability in voiding data. Above 50 cm H_2O, i.e., group IV, all patients are definitely obstructed, and minor changes following therapy are of little interest because they indicate only a slight difference in obstruction, where a clinically relevant change in outflow condition would be related to a drop in pressure of at least 25 cm H_2O. Above 100 cm H_2O, i.e., grade VI, all patients are drastically obstructed, and we see no clinical sense in subclassifying drastic obstruction. Any meaningful therapy in this group must reduce outflow conditions at least 50 cm H_2O, and minor changes are hardly of interest. Furthermore, in our clinic the percentage of patients above group VI, i.e., 150 cm H_2O voiding and opening pressure, is negligibly small, and their clinical classification needs no further differentation.

◀────────────────────────────

Fig. 4a, b. Various features and results from the clinical application of the „linear PURR". **a** *Upper panel, solid lines,* a typical obstructed voiding pattern of BPH; *broken lines,* a good result from surgery. *Small lines,* the critical points that must be identified for the „linear PURR", which are the pressure at peak flow and the minimum pressure at which flow is possible, equivalent to the minimum urethral opening pressure (p_{muo}). It is necessary to correct for the time delay in the flow rate recording, and the corresponding lines on the flow curve are therefore shifted here for 1 s earlier with respect to the pressure curve. At the termination of voiding a correct identification of the lowest pressure requires the elimination of the last few milliliters which leave the distal urethra after the prostatic urethra is already closed (here, after 39 s for the obstructed tracing and after 30 s for the normal one). These points are transferred to the pressure/flow diagram in Figure **b** and result in the characteristic linear PURR with the grading IV/N = obstructed/normal detrusor, and I/N = normalized outflow with unchanged detrusor strength. **a** *Lower panel,* other relevant features of the linear PURR. *Solid line* typical for a constrictive obstruction and untypical for BPH. This is the reason why it does not lead to a clear classification in this pressure/flow diagram **(b)** which is adapted for compressive obstruction as in BPH. *Broken line* (**a**, *lower panel*) shows a voiding pattern which by its flow rate curve is often misinterpreted as confirming obstructive BPH. The linear PURR and the pressure/flow diagram demonstrate clear that this is a completely unobstructed bladder outlet which, in combination with a very weak detrusor, results in poor voiding function

Grading Detrusor Function

Voiding is a „two-dimensional" balance between outflow and detrusor function, and all information about this mechanical balance is contained implicitly in the pressure/flow curves. Thus, in a similar simplifying approach as for the outlet it is possible roughly to assess detrusor contraction strength with the linear PURR. The top end of the linear PURR is the data point of maximum flow rate and peak flow pressure and thus represents maximal contractile power for the detrusor. A line for grading same muscle power would need to follow a hyperbolic line (see Fig. 1), according to typical behavior of the active muscle [11, 17, 18]. As for the outflow conditions, it is possible to obtain meaningful results, again by using a linear approximation. This is definitely adequate for a rough classification into the four categories of very weak, weak, normal, and strong detrusor contraction function. Additionally, it must be taken into account that detrusor contraction strength is rather variable, that it depends on the bladder filling volume as indicated by the dependence of peak flow on volume, and that it is of rather limited clinical relevance. Diagnostically, the outflow conditions are definitely of prime importance because they can be treated, but there is no effective therapeutic approach to enhance a weak detrusor contraction. Lastly, both outflow conditions and detrusor strength are aspects of the same mechanical balance, which means that when one term (grade of obstruction) is defined, the other term is obvious. A normal outlet produces a flow rate according to the detrusor strength, and the combination of a very weak (VW) detrusor with a severe obstruction (grade V) simply cannot result in voiding. It is very interesting to see how close the shift of the tip of the linear PURR follows the lines of same detrusor strength when pre- and postoperative voiding studies are analyzed for the same patient (see Fig. 4).

Defining Obstruction

The most important step for the clinical application of an analytical concept such as the pressure/flow diagram is the question of how this diagram and the derived grading of outflow obstruction and detrusor contraction strength can be validated. This question is related to my introductory remarks and again points out the need for an extensive discussion of the rather vague and often obscure use of the term „obstruction" in urology.

As the urodynamic data are the only objective, measurable, reproducible, i.e., quantitative, data on bladder voiding function, it becomes obvious that no other objective data on obstruction are available which could be used to calibrate the pressure/flow diagram. The use of this diagram for retrospective data analysis from patients undergoing transurethral resection of the prostate makes clear that the traditional data do lead to different results. There is no clear and definite correlation in BPH between the urodynamic measure of obstructed function and any of the standard obstruction parameters. Although the relation between many of these parameters and the urodynamic result may be statistically significant, it is still clear that a significant proportion (20%–30%) of patients undergoing prostatic surgery according to traditional concepts are definitely unobstructed urodynamically [19, 23, 24]. Thus, clinical data which could be used to validate the objective urodynamic grading are not available.

Considering the imprecise nature of these data and the high placebo effect of any treatment of symptoms and signs of „obstructive BPH", it is clear that only a blinded study with the indication for prostatectomies based on the urodynamic grading of obstruction would provide a useful data base.

Therefore, I have used an indirect approach to identify a border between „obstructed" and „unobstructed" which can be used clinically, and which has a potential for scientific research. If we compare the urodynamic data from patients before and after prostatectomy, we can clearly describe and quantify the typical change after surgery on objective voiding function. Using the same type of data and the same analytical approach with the pressure/flow diagram, we can distinguish those urodynamic values which are typically changed by surgery from those which remain unchanged after surgery. When we make such an objective comparative analysis, we find that only patients with grade II show a definite change after surgery. This allows the specific surgical definition of bladder outflow obstruction, i.e., grade 0/I unobstructed and grade II and higher increasingly obstructed, which is of clinical value (Fig. 5).

This definition implies neither that asymptomatic voiding with grade II or higher requires surgical intervention, nor that symptomatic patients with grad I or 0 cannot improve symptomatically from surgery. It means only that objective voiding function will not be better and may be worse after surgery of grade 0/I, and that patients with grade II most likely will be better after surgery. Further, the probability and extent of urodynamic, i.e., improvement in voiding function, increases with the preoperative degree of obstruction.

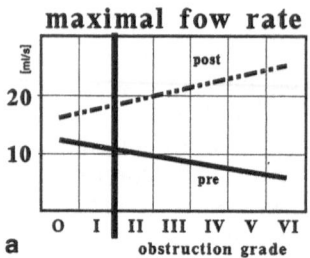

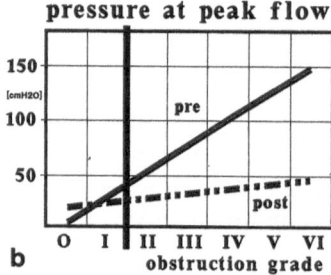

Fig. 5a, b. The traditional urodynamic values of maximum flow rate (**a**) and maximum pressure at peak flow (**b**) are classified according to the obstruction grade from the pressure/flow diagram and compared for pre- and postoperative voiding. Here we use linear regression to analyze the data reported in Langen et al. (this volume). Both panels show clearly that the improvement in voiding function after transurethral resection of the prostate depend on the grade of obstruction. The change in voiding pressure shows that only in patients with at least grade II before surgery is a significant decrease in voiding pressure found

Scientific Application

We have used the urodynamic assessment of obstruction in a large number of patients, and the pressure/flow diagram has now been used for grading more than 1000 voiding studies (see Langen et al., this volume). We have also used the diagram for retrospective analysis of a number of urodynamic studies of new treatment modalities such as drugs, balloon dilatation, and thermotherapy. The results from this extensive experience is that objective urodynamic grading deviates from the clinical judgement in all studies, and that particularly the uroflow as a single urodynamic parameter is almost useless because of its low specificity for bladder outflow obstruction.

In summary, we find with the pressure/flow diagram that the objective decrease in bladder outflow obstruction is minor or nonexistent from alpha-blockers [26], cannot be verified for thermotherapy, and is the clear exception after balloon dilatation [19].

Conclusion

It is clear from our data that the traditional concepts and common use today of the term obstruction in urology are not based on objective data. For the most common „obstructive" disease (BPH) it is very obvious that approximately 20% – 30% of patients treated today by prostatectomy are not objectively obstructed before and thus cannot improve in voiding function ([23]; Langen et al., this volume). From this point of view, the real need for or benefit from surgery remains unclear in these unobstructed patients. The majority of dissatisfied patients are in the unobstructed group; however, the majority of unobstructed and urodynamically unimproved patients are nevertheless satisfied with the result of transurethral resection of the prostate.

From the fact that the urodynamic results are in controversy to the traditional clinical parameters, it is commonly concluded, that urodynamics is unreliable and unspecific, that the urodynamic data analysis is wrong or that urodynamics is not even measuring the real function. My conclusion is just the opposite, that the scientific methodology and the objective data from urodynamics must be used to reevaluate and reestablish the traditional clinical concepts of obstruction on a sound basis.

References

1. Abrams PH, Griffiths DJ (1979) The assesment of prostatic obstruction from urodynamic measurements and from residual urine. Br J Urol 51:129–134
2. Abrams PH, Schäfer W (1984) Urodynamic aspects of detrusor mechanics and contractility. World J urol 2:174–180
3. Bruskewitz R, Jensen KM-E, Iversen P, Madsen PO (1983) The relevance of minimum urethral resistance in prostatism. J Urol 129:769–771
4. Gammelgaard PA, Andersen JT, Meyhoff HH (1983) Clinical significance of urodynamic measurements. In: Hinman F Jr (ed) Benign prostatic hypertrophy. Springer, Berlin Heidelberg New York, pp 502–506
5. Griffiths DJ (1980) Urodynamics. Hilger, Bristol (Medical physics handbooks, vol 4)
6. Griffiths DJ, van Mastrigt R, Bosch R (1989) Quantification of urethral resistance and bladder function during voiding, with special reference to the effects of prostate size reduction on urethral obstruction due to benign prostatic hyperplasia. Neurourol Urodyn 8:17–27
7. International Continence Society (1987) Urodynamic equipment: technical aspects. J Med Eng Technol 11:57–64
8. Lutzeyer W. Hannappel J, Schäfer W (1983) Sequential events in prostatic obstruction. In: Hinman F Jr (ed) Benign prostatic hypertrophy. Springer, Berlin Heidelberg New York, pp 693–700
9. Melchior H, Jaschke W (1983) Urodynamic interpretation of symptoms. In: Hinman F Jr (ed) Benign prostatic hypertrophy. Springer, Berlin Heidelberg New York, pp 627–641

10. Meyhoff HH, Gleason DM, Bottaccini MR (1989) The effects of transurethral resection on the urodynamics of prostatism. J Urol 142:785–789
11. Schäfer W (1983) Detrusor as the energy source of micturition. In: Hinman F Jr (ed) Benign prostatic hypertrophy. Springer, Berlin Heidelberg New York, pp 450–469
12. Schäfer W (1983) The contribution of the bladder outlet to the relation between pressure and flow rate during micturition. In: Hinman F Jr (ed) Benign prostatic hypertrophy. Springer, Berlin Heidelberg New York, pp 470–496
13. Schäfer W (1985) Urethral resistance? Urodynamic concepts of physiological and pathological bladder outlet function during voiding. Neurourol Urodyn 4:161–201
14. Schäfer W (1987) Mechanics of normal and obstructed micturition. In: Benign prostatic hyperplasia, vol II. NIH, Bethesda, pp 211–220 (National Institutes of Health publication no. 87-2881)
15. Schäfer W (1989) Editorial comment. In: Spangberg A, Terio H, Engberg A, Ask P (1989) Quantification of urethral function based on Griffiths' model of flow through elastic tubes. Neurourol Urodyn 8:44–50
16. Schäfer W (1990) Principles and clinical application of advanced urodynamic analysis of voiding function. Urol Clin North Am 17:553–566
17. Schäfer W (1991) Analysis of active detrusor function during voiding with the bladder working function. Neurourol Urodyn 10:19–35
18. Schäfer W (1991) Detrusor muscle mechanics in clinical urodynamics. In: Siroky MB, Krane RB (eds) Clinical neuro-urology, 2nd edn. Little and Brown, Boston
19. Schäfer W (1992) Urodynamik bei benigner Prostatahyperplasie. In: Rutishauser G, Vahlensieck W (eds) Benigne Prostatopathien. Thieme, Stuttgart, pp 134–149
20. Schäfer W, Abrams PH (1979) The voiding patterns of adult enuretics. Proceedings of the International Continence Society, Rome, 4–6 Oct. 1979, pp 227–230
21. Schäfer W, Fischer B, Meyhoff HH, Lutzeyer W (1981) Urethral resistance during voiding: the passive urethral resistance relation, PURR. Proceedings of the International Continence Society, Lund, 3–5 Sept. 1981, pp 31–33
22. Schäfer W, Noppeney R, Rübben H, Lutzeyer W (1988) The value of free flow rate and pressure/flow-studies in the routine investigation of BPH patients. Neurourol Urodyn 7:219–221
23. Schäfer W, Rübben H, Noppeney R, Deutz F-J (1989) Obstructed and unobstructed prostatic obstruction. A plea for urodynamic objectivation of bladder outflow obstruction in benign prostatic hyperplasia. World J Urol 6:198–203
24. Schäfer W, Waterbär F, Langen PH, Deutz F-J (1989) A simplified graphic procedure for detailed analysis of detrusor and outlet function during voiding. Neurourol Urodyn 8:405–407
25. Schäfer W, Langen PH, Thörner M (1990) The real pressure/flow-relation during obstructed voiding. Neurourol Urodyn 9:423–425
26. Schäfer W, Hermanns R, Langen PH, Abrams PH, Chappel CR, Stott M (1991) Urodynamic analysis of drug effects on bladder voiding function: statistical significance and clinical relevance. Neurourol Urodyn 10:288–289
27. Spangberg A, Terio H, Engberg A, Ask P (1989) Quantification of urethral function based on Griffiths' model of flow through elastic tubes. Neurourol Urodyn 8:29–52
28. Turner Warwick R (1983) The symptoms of bladder outlet obstruction. In: Hinman F Jr (ed) Benign prostatic hypertrophy. Springer, Berlin Heidelberg New York, pp 701–705

Operative Treatment

When Should Open Prostatectomy Be Performed?

G. Hubmer, T. Colombo, and M. Rauchenwald[1]

Introduction

Transurethral resection of the prostate (TUR) is the method of choice in the management of benign prostatic hyperplasia (BPH). This is true for adenomas with an estimated weight of up to 60 g. However, is TUR also the best procedure for adenomas larger than 60 g?

Many urologists perform transvesical or retropubic open prostatectomy for prostatic adenomas weighing more than 50–60 g. If the right moment is chosen for open prostatectomy in such a case, this operation is superior to TUR. The cumulative percentage of patients undergoing a second prostatectomy is substantially higher after transurethral than after open prostatectomy (12% versus 4.5%). Investigations on this subject were conducted by Roos et al. in 1989 [6], and the data are based on more than 50 000 patients in Denmark, the United Kingdom, and Canada. A distinct difference was seen in long-term mortality, with an elevated rate for TUR patients compared to those receiving open prostatectomy. The follow-up periods were 3 months, 1, 5, and 8 years after the operation. Only at the first postoperative examination after 90 days was the mortality rate for TUR patients in Denmark between aged 75–84 years slightly lower than that for open prostatectomy. In all the other age groups in all three countries the open operation was more favorable regarding long-term mortality and probability for a second prostatectomy after 1, 3, and 8 years.

Which patients should be considered for open prostatectomy? First, patients aged up to 65 years with an prostatic adenoma weighing more than 50–60 g, would benefit by the lower risk of second prostatectomy. Further advantages are due to the large amount of tissue removed in a short operating time, more radical tissue removal, and low rate of postoperative contracture of the bladder neck, ranging from 0.9% to 1.1%

---

[1] Chirurgische Universitätsklinik, Urologische Abteilung, Auenbrugger Platz 15, A-8036 Graz, Austria

[1, 3, 4]. Disadvantages of open prostatectomy include: higher perioperative mortality, ranging from 2% to 3.1% [1, 3, 4] compared to TUR (0.0% −2%) [5], higher risk of postoperative bleeding, the possibility of wound infection, and the risk of urinary infection by long-term indwelling urethral catheter.

We would like to call attention to two problems, those of urinary infection and postoperative blood loss. The incidence of postoperative urinary infection can be reduced by modifications in the open prostatectomy. From 1967 to 1976, 350 patients with prostatic adenomas were managed by the catheterless method of suprapubic transvesical prostatectomy. The aim of this technique was the avoidance of the bacterial urinary infection due to the indwelling catheter and of the bladder neck stricture [3].

Method and Results

The adenoma is enucleated digitally, and the prostatic cavity is packed with a warm, moist pack for a period of 5−10min. The prostatic arteries and other bleeding vessels are controlled by sutures placed especially at 5 and 7 o'clock position. The bladder neck remains open widely. Only extremely wide bladder necks are narrowed by anterior sutures. Two 12-F Redi-Vac suction drains are inserted into the prostatic cavity across the bladder, so that one-third of the perforations are in the prostatic fossa and two-thirds in the bladder (Fig. 1).

The drains are brought out through the bladder wall on each side of the cystotomy and through the abdominal wall using the spike introducer. The wound is closed with a prevesical drain. Diuresis is stimulated by furosemide. Postoperative care is simple. Full or badly work-

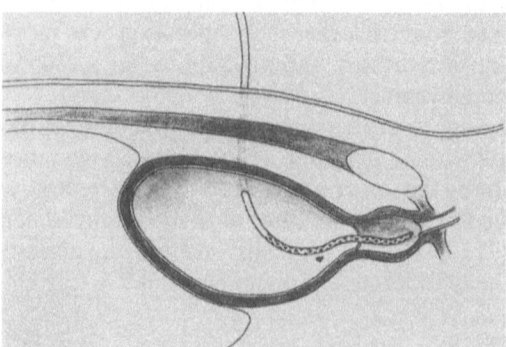

Fig. 1. Position of Redi-Vac drainage after prostatectomy

Table 1. Complication in 350 cases of catheterless prostatectomy. (From [4])

	n	%
Mortality	7	2.0
Severe postoperative hemorrhage	10	2.8
Suprapubic fistula (controlled by catheter)	12	3.4
Epididymitis	3	0.9
Contracture of bladder neck	3	0.9
Chronic urinary infection	14	4.0

ing vacuum bottles are changed. Obstruction of the system with blood clots may occur within the first few hours. A good diuresis generally avoids this complication. The first drain is removed on the third postoperative day, the second on the sixth or seventh day. Some patients may pass urine per urethram although the drainage system works sufficiently; however, this occurs mainly due to detrusor spasms.

The functional results have been excellent. Only three patients have developed moderate stricture of the bladder neck (Table 1). Eighty-five patients came to the operation without infection and these patients were not treated with antibiotics; in this group only ten developed a significant urinary infection after surgery (Table 2).

The second problem is the handling of intra- and postoperative hemorrhage. This can be avoided substantially by the application of fibrin sealant [2] and other blood-stanching methods, for instance, tamponade with balloon catheter or gauze strip (which must be removed!), special suture technique (purse-string suture) for self-tamponade of the prostatic fossa, continuous suction drainage, operation under controlled hypotension, or systemic use of hemostatic agents.

Because of the increasing role of TUR in the management of BPH a decreasing number of patients are being operated on by open surgery. With about ten open prostatectomies per year, this operation has become a rare procedure at our clinic. At the beginning of 1991, however, we resumed the catheterless open prostatectomy in a modified

Table 2. Antibiotics and urinary infection in 350 patients. (From [4])

	n	%
With antibiotics	265	
Without antibiotics	85	
No postoperative bacteriuria	48	57
Significant bacteriuria	10	11
Not checked (asymptomatic)	27	32

way using fibrin glue (Tissucol) as a sealant of the prostatic fossa [2]. This fibrin glue is applied in the prostatic cavity and pressed against the capsule by an inflated 50-ml balloon of an indwelling catheter for 10 min. The catheter is then removed. Only one 16-F Redi-Vac drain is used. Postoperative blood loss seems less, and negative consequences of this technique have so far not been observed.

Conclusion

Despite the almost exclusive use of TUR in the management of BPH over the past two decades one should not forget the technique of open transvesical prostatectomy as a potentially effective tool in selected cases. Particularly younger patients with very large prostatic adenomas are benefited by this. This is due particularly to the low incidence of relapse after open prostatectomy, as reported by Roos et al. [6]. This seems to be the crucial point in determining the operative procedure for younger patients with large adenomas. The decision for open operation is made much easier if one uses all the improvements which have been made in open operating techniques, in particular various blood-stanching methods. As another modification of open prostatectomy, the catheterless method spares the patient substantial discomfort. For adenomas weighing more than 60 g the short operating time is an additional advantage. Lastly, open prostatectomy should be performed only by fully trained urologists who master this technique of operation.

References

1. Bollmann J, Zingg E (1976) Retropubic prostatectomy. In: Marberger H, Haschek H, Schirmer HKA, Colston JAC, Witkin E (eds) Prostatic disease. Liss, New York, p 59
2. Gasser G, Mossig G, Fischer M, Eidler R, Kläring W, Lurf H (1983) Modifikation der suprapubischen Prostatektomie unter Verwendung eines biologischen Klebeverfahrens. Wien. Klin Wochenschr 95:399–403
3. Hohenfellner R (1976) Suprapubic prostatectomy. In: Marberger H, Haschek H, Schirmer HKA, Colston JAC, Witkin E (eds) Prostatic disease. Liss, New York, p 49
4. Hubmer G, Lipsky H, Petritsch P, Eppich F (1977) Prostatectomy with a no-catheter technique. Br J Urol 49:315–317
5. Mebust WK, Holtgrewe HL, Cockett ATK, Peters PC, Writing Committee (1989) Transurethral prostatectomy: immediate and postoperative complications. A cooperative study of 13 participating institutions evaluating 3.885 patients. J Urol 141:243–247
6. Roos NP, Wennberg JE, Malenka DJ, Fisher ES, McPherson K, Andersen TF, Cohen MM, Ramsey E (1989) Mortality and reoperation after open and transurethral resection of the prostate for benign prostatic hyperplasia. N Engl J Med 320:1120–1124

Retropubic Transcervical Prostatectomy Without Catheter as a Modification of the Millin Technique

H. Baur and J. E. Altwein[1]

Introduction

In comparison to the commonly performed transurethral adenomectomy the retropubic method of prostatectomy has gained new importance recently. This is due to the extensive studies of Roos et al. [7], who demonstrated that the rate of necessary reoperations was four to six times more frequent after transurethral adenomectomy than with retropubic prostatectomy. In this study the average weight of the transurethrally treated prostates was 66 g. Most urologists, however, prefer the retropubic adenomectomy only for heavier prostates.

Since this operation was first performed by Fuller in 1895 [2], one of the major problems of adenomectomy by the retropubic approach has been management of the inevitable bleeding [3]. Many studies have demonstrated the necessity of a bleeding prophylaxis, since especially elderly men with cardiopulmonary risk factors are vitally endangered by the blood loss. The standard procedure for suprapubic transvesical adenomectomy is the technique of Harris [4] and Hryntschak [5], which prevents secondary bleeding by a special sewing method of the prostatic fossa. Harris tried to avoid the problem of fossal stenosis − one of the major disadvantages of this technique − by fixating bladder mucosa at the lowest point of the surgical capsule (so-called deep retrigonization). The retropubic approach for adenomectomy allows a better view of the prostatic fossa and thus a more subtle removal of very large and even small adenomas. This technique was carried out for the first time in 1909 by van Stockum [7] as a so-called „extravesical" adenomectomy. Millin in 1945 rendered this procedure the standard technique of the retropubic approach for adenomectomy [6].

[1] Krankenhaus der Barmherzigen Brüder, Urologische Abteilung, Romanstraße 93, W-8000 München 19, FRG

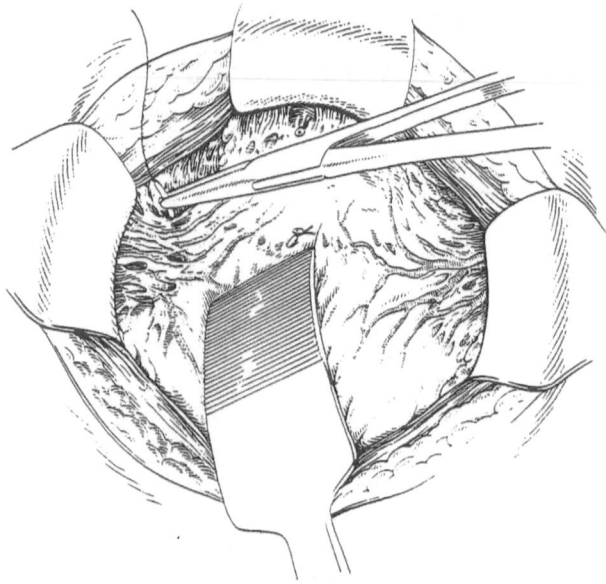

Fig. 1. The retropubic region is exposed, the ventral prostate capsule is freed of fat tissue, the vena dorsalis penis ligated and transected. The vesicoprostatic bundle is ligated by a 1/0 chrom cat mass suture (From [1] with permission)

To prevent nosocomial infections operative procedures without catheter drainages from the urinary tract should be prefered. This is especially true for retropubic adenomectomy. We use a modified retropubic technique with the following features:

- prophylactic hemostasis by ligating the vesicoprostatic vascular bundle,
- large excision of the ventral prostatic capsule and the ventral bladder neck commissure,
- circumcision of the bladder outlet,
- reduction in the volume of the fossa by purse-string sutures, and deep retrigonization.

With this modified technique of Millin [6] we performed 3000 retropubic adenomectomies between 1970 and 1990. Of these operations 85% were effective primarily without placing a transurethral catheter. With an average patient age of 70 years and an average adenoma weight of 64 g, our postoperative lethality was 1.5%. Secondary bleeding was noted in 6.2%; secondary operations such as transurethral coagulation or resection with fossal clearing were performed in 3.0% [1].

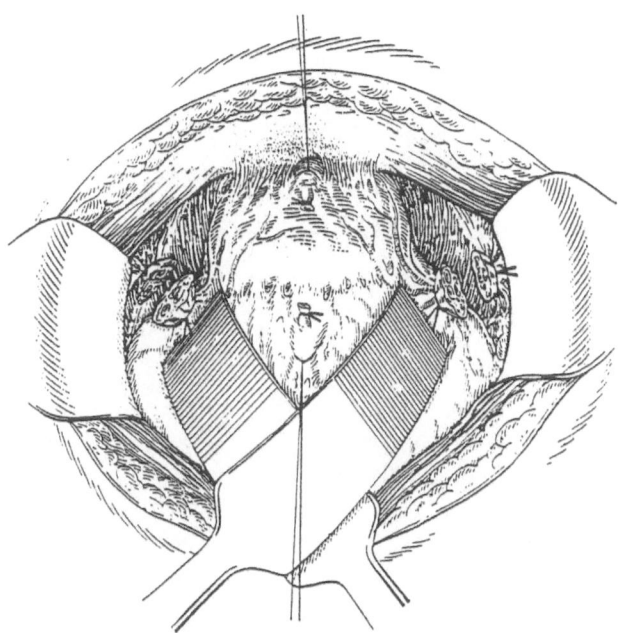

Fig. 2. Exposition of bladder outlet by means of so-called Kader retractors. The distal capsule suture in the region of the puboprostatic ligaments and the proximal suture of the bladder outlet are ligated. The vesicoprostatic bundles are ligated and transected on both sides (From [1] with permission)

Technique

Place the patient in supine position with slightly abducted and lowered legs. Open the retropubic space by means of a Pfannenstiel incision (Fig. 1). Perform the intrapelvic vasectomy in the junction between the peritoneum and the vena iliaca externa as prophylaxis against epididymitis. Expose the bladder neck and prostate (Fig. 2). Ligate and transect the vena dorsalis penis. To prevent hemostasis secure the vesicoprostatic vessels on both sides at the lateral prostate wall with a 1/0 chromcat suture (so-called Grégoir's suture) [3]. With sexually active patients these sutures should not be applied so as not to injure the neurovascular bundle.

Place a fixation suture cranially and caudally from the planned oval excision of the prostate capsule. Lay the distal suture as near as possible to the puboprostatic ligaments. Identify the ureteral orifices by administering indigo carmine intravenously (Fig. 3). Open the bladder outlet with a small horizontal incision, and excise the ventral prostate

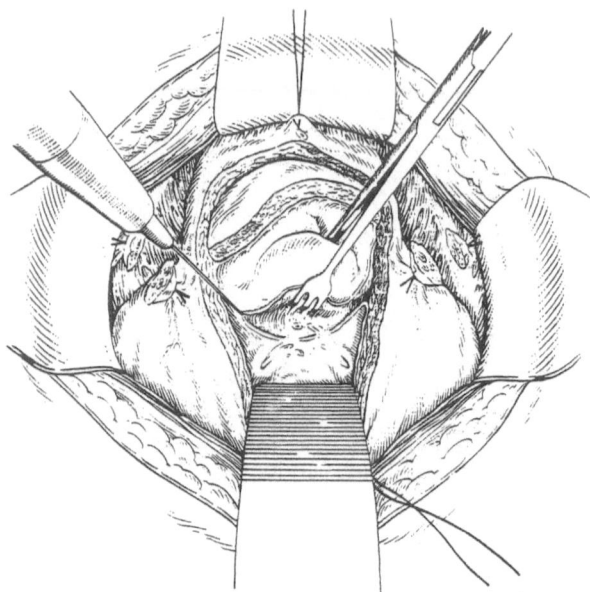

Fig. 3. Circumcision of the adenoma distal from the ureteral orifices. Situs immediately before the digital enucleation of the adenoma. Control of position and function of the ureteral orifices by intravenous indigo carmine (From [1] with permission)

capsule ovally (Fig. 4). Use additional sutures and electrocoagulation as needed to control bleeding. Peritomize the adenoma distally from the ureteral orifices, and digitally enucleate it after breaking the urethra anteriorly (Fig. 5).

Cut the urethra at the level of the apex (Fig. 6). The more parts of ventral prostate capsule are resected, the better one can see the apical region. After enucleation inspect the fossa, and control complete adenoma removal. Apply purse-string sutures for final control of bleeding. Place a 1/0 chrom cat sutures as far distally and dorsally as possible through the prostate capsule together with the bladder wall about one-half in. laterally from the ureteral orifices. Thereby it is possible to put the bladder floor into a caudal position and simultaneously to reduce the volume of the fossa.

With the purse-string sutures applied, bleeding can normally no longer be observed. Now the retrigonization can be achieved easily. Sew the trigonum with a 3/0 catgut interrupted suture as near as possible to the collicle and repeat this procedure with bladder mucosa until

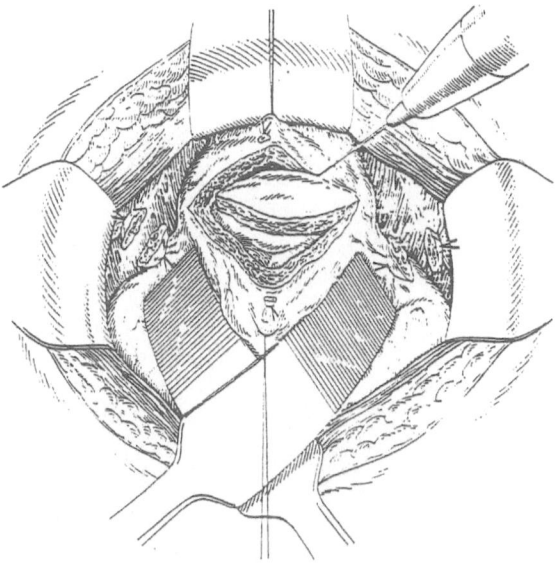

Fig. 4. Broad partial excision of the ventral prostate capsule and oval circumcision of the bladder outlet with the electrocauter between the preliminary sutures (From [1] with permission)

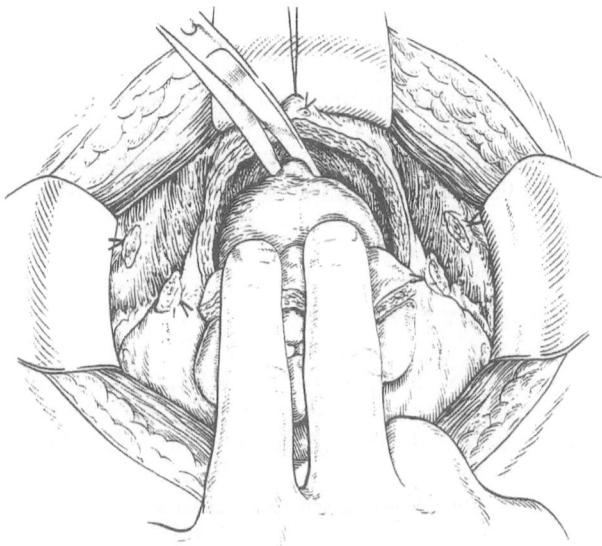

Fig. 5. Sharp separation of the adenoma from the distal urethra made possible by prior broad excision of the ventral prostate capsule (From [1] with permission)

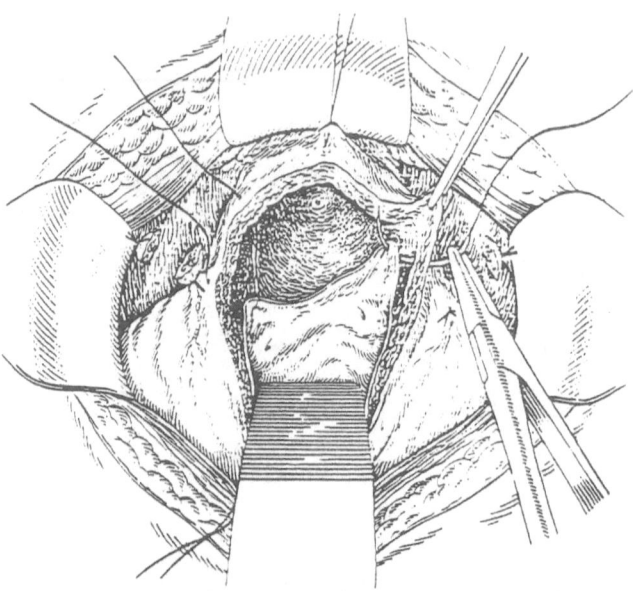

Fig. 6. Situs after enucleation. The 1/0 chrom cat purse-string sutures are brought into position on both sides to reduce the volume of the fossa and transpose the trigonum (From [1] with permission)

a smooth and wide junction between bladder and fossa is created (Fig. 7).

For a cystostomy apply an 18-F catheter extravulnarily for temporary urine deviation. Close the prostate capsule with 1/0 chrom cat interrupted sutures (Fig. 8). Drain the periprostatic region with a 30-F silicon tube. Control complete hemostasis by irrigating the bladder via cystostomy.

Secondary Treatment

The 18-F cystostomy commonly remains in situ for 5 days. For all patients without cardiovascular risk factors induce a forced diuresis by generously substituting body fluid, thus irrigating the bladder physiologically. On day 6 after the operation close and remove the cystostomy when voiding without residual urine is possible.

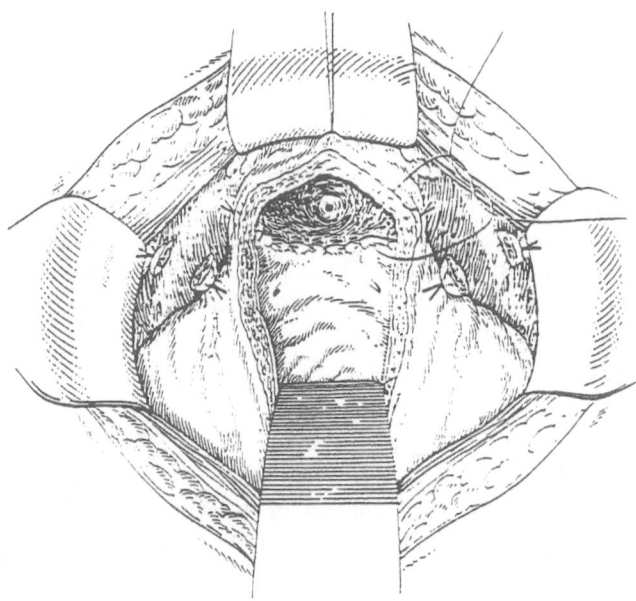

Fig. 7. So-called deep retrigonization to create a wide nonobstructive junction from the fossa to the bladder (From [1] with permission)

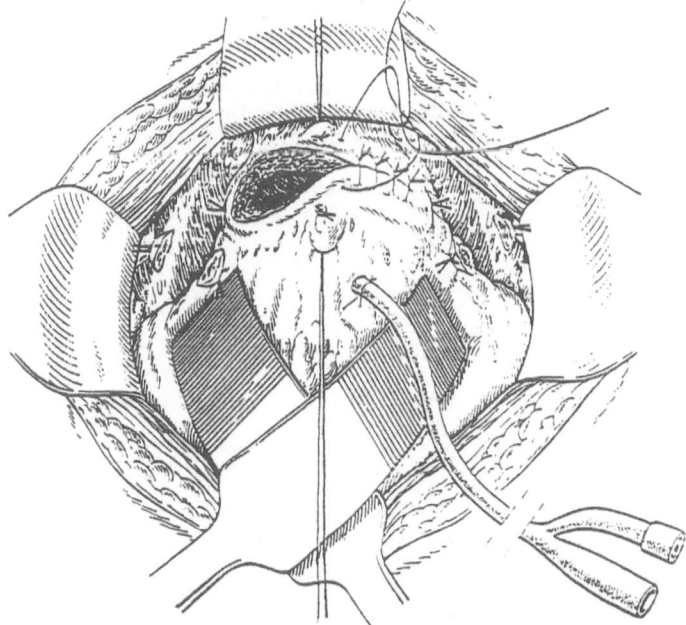

Fig. 8. Closure of the ventral prostate capsule with 1/0 chrom cat interrupted sutures. Cystostomy 18-F in position (From [1] with permission)

Discussion

The patient due for adenomectomy has a high risk for infections by ob structive voiding. The aim of any surgical treatment should always be to discharge the primarily noninfected patient without causing a newly acquired infection, especially without the dangerous polyresistant hospital germs. Furthermore, the imminent danger of postoperative urethral strictures should be reduced by avoiding tamponating transurethral balloon catheters. The combination of the above technical procedures makes it possible to avoid routinely transurethral catheters after adenomectomy and thereby to decrease the rate of infection and strictures.

References

1. Baur H, Altwein JE, Schneider W (1990) Retropubische Adenomektomie der Prostata. Akt Urol 21 [Suppl Operative Techniken] I–VIII
2. Fuller E (1895) Six successful and successive cases of prostatectomy. J Gut Genitourine Dis 13:229–233
3. Grégoir W (1969) Heostatic adenomectomy. Urol Int 24:426–438
4. Harris SH (1929) Suprapubic prostatectomy with closure. J Urol 1:285–289
5. Hryntschak T (1951) Die suprapubische Prostatektomie mit primärem Blasenverschluß nach eigener Methode. Maudrich, Vienna
6. Millin T (1945) Retropubic prostatectomy: a new extravesical technique. Lancet 2:693–696
7. Roos NP, Wenneberg JE, Malenka DJ, Fisher ES, McPherson K, Folmer-Anderson T, Cohen MM, Ramsey E (1989) Mortality and reoperation after open and transurethral resection of the prostate for benign prostatic hyperplasia. N Engl J Med 320:1120–1124
8. von Stockum W (1909) Prostatectomia suprapubica extravesicalis. Zentralbl Chir 36:41–43

Video-Guided Transurethral Resection: Raising the Gold Standard

P. Faul[1]

Transurethral resection (TUR) of the prostate is still the gold standard for surgical treatment of prostate adenoma. In our clinic, for example, 96% of all adenomas of the prostate requiring surgery are resected transurethrally. TUR has a high success rate and is associated with improvements in flow rate, bladder emptying, and quality of life [11].

Efforts to treat prostate adenoma conservatively, using less invasive procedures, are ushering in a new era in the therapy of benign prostatic hyperplasia. A major new development in this direction is video TUR, the extension to transurethral resection of the video technology already used by gynecologists, orthopedists, and, more recently, general surgeons [2, 8, 13, 20, 21].

Astoundingly, in urology, the leading endoscopic specialty, only a few individual surgeons have performed endoscopic surgery with video guidance [1, 15–17, 22–25]. The first report in the German-language literature appeared only recently [5]. Now, however, integration of the video technique with the use of smaller, lighter, high-resolution minichip cameras is opening up new perspectives for endoscopic surgery.

Apparatus and Method

All operations on the prostate are currently performed with low-pressure irrigation (LP-TUR) using a continuous-flow resectoscope; if the estimated weight of the adenoma exceeds 40 g, suprapubic, paracentesis of the bladder is carried out as well. This ensures optimal flow, an absolute precondition for adequate video quality. The advantages of LP-TUR over high-pressure irrigation (HP-TUR) are well known [4, 7,

---

[1] Stadtkrankenhaus Memmingen, Urologische Abteilung,
W-8940 Memmingen, FRG

12, 18, 19, 24]. In the case of transurethral resection of large adenomas (estimated weight exceeding 70 g), intraoperative autotransfusion may be carried out if necessary [6].

We use the following apparatus for video TUR:

- A 33-cm monitor (Sony PVM 1442)
- A steering device
- A high -intensity 400-W halogen light source with electronic brightness regulation via video signal
- A VHS video recorder

The apparatus is accomodated on a specially designed cart (Fig. 1). Our power source is an Erbe generator (Erbotom ACC 430 no. A 1013).

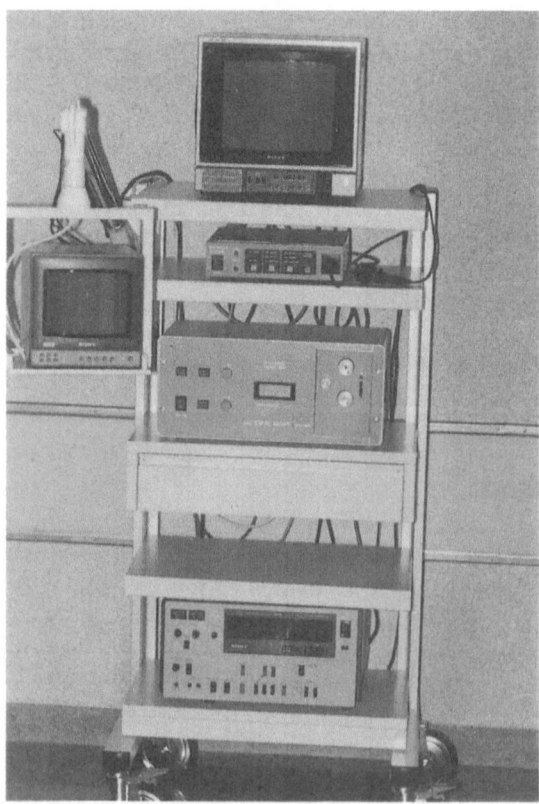

Fig. 1. Video apparatus on specially designed cart

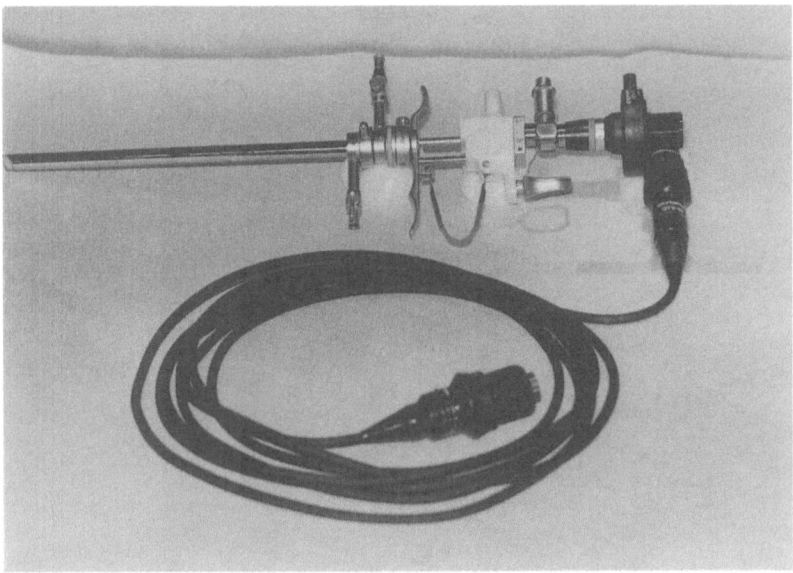

Fig. 2. Olympus resectoscope and minichip camera

The minicamera (Olympus OTV S-2) is coupled to the eyepiece of the continuous-flow resectoscope (Olympus) with an adapter (type ARTF/2) (Fig. 2). For reasons of sterility the camera and cable are sheated in plastic. The whole system is sterilizable. The video images are shown on two monitors. The smaller of these, the working monitor, is mounted on a swivel arm from the video cart and positioned over that patient. The surgeon watches this screen with both eyes, and it provides the only orientation for positioning of the cutting loop during resection. Others (e.g., anesthetist, assistants, and other staff) can follow the transurethral procedure on the second, larger monitor.

Clinical Significance of Video TUR

The surgeon's comfortable seated position and the binocular observation of the monitor (Fig. 3) considerably reduce eye strain and obviate the constant contortions that are necessary to look through the eyepiece in conventional TUR (Fig. 4). The „TUR surgeon's syndrome" – acute and chronic symptoms in the cervical and lumbar spine – is largely eliminated. The surgeon tires less quickly and does not often need a break. As a result, the procedure has to be interrupted so

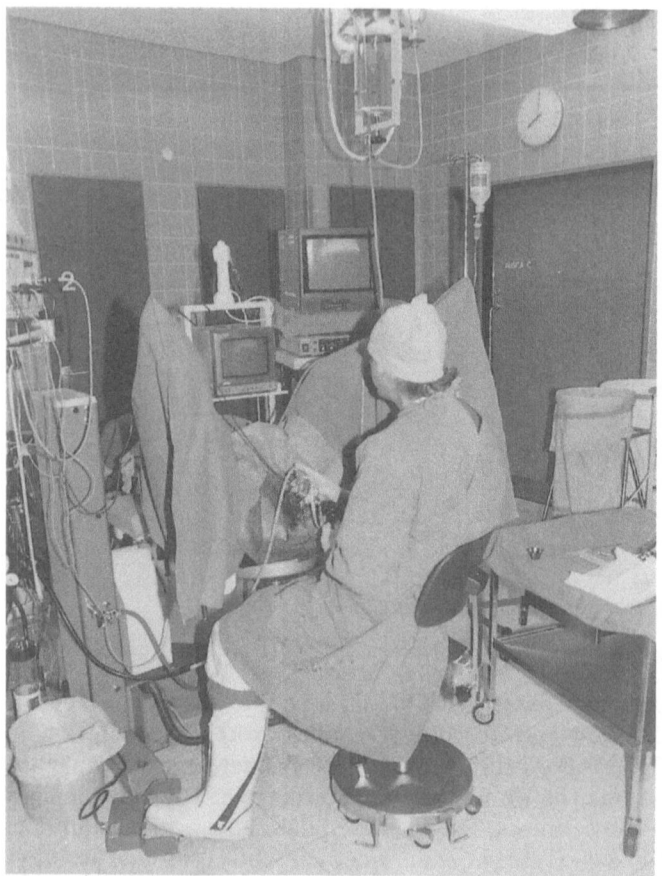

Fig. 3. Surgeon's comfortable position during video TUR

that the continuous-flow resectoscope can be used just to remove the debris of resection; with a resection weight of 20–30 g only one or two such interruptions are required.

We carried out 470 video-guided TUR procedures between June 1989 and October 1991. Resection time went down considerably in the 1.5 years to the time of writing, with the tissue removal rate increasing from 0.8 g/min to 1.5 g/min.

With the conventional resection technique, contamination with urine is frequent because of the direct contact between the surgeon's eye and the eyepiece and sheath of the resectoscope. The operator runs the risk of contracting bacterial infections such as tuberculosis or viral

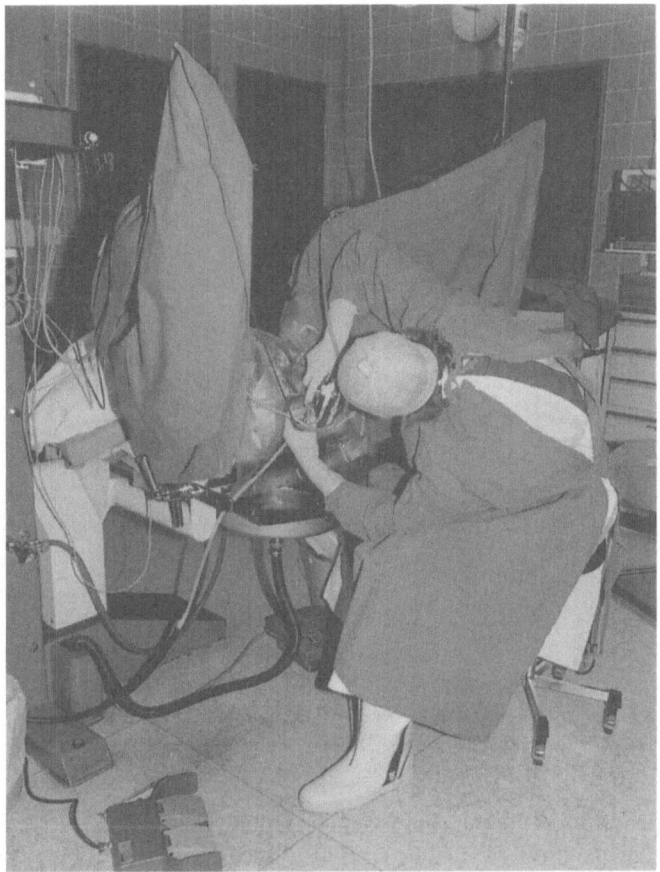

Fig. 4. Surgeon's contorted position during conventional TUR

diseases such as AIDS or hepatitis B [10]. McNicholas et al. [14] reported a 46% rate of infection of the eye or face among surgeons operating on a total of 99 patients. Findings such as these led Davies and Harrison [3] to recommend that surgeons wear spectacles during TUR – a measure that becomes superfluous with video TUR.

In the past severe problems have been encountered in teaching TUR, which usually takes place in darkness. With the hitherto available optical systems teachers have found it difficult to demonstrate the transurethral procedure and students have had difficulty in following the operation. The advent of the video technique enables TUR to taught much more effectively. The visibility of the monitor to all those

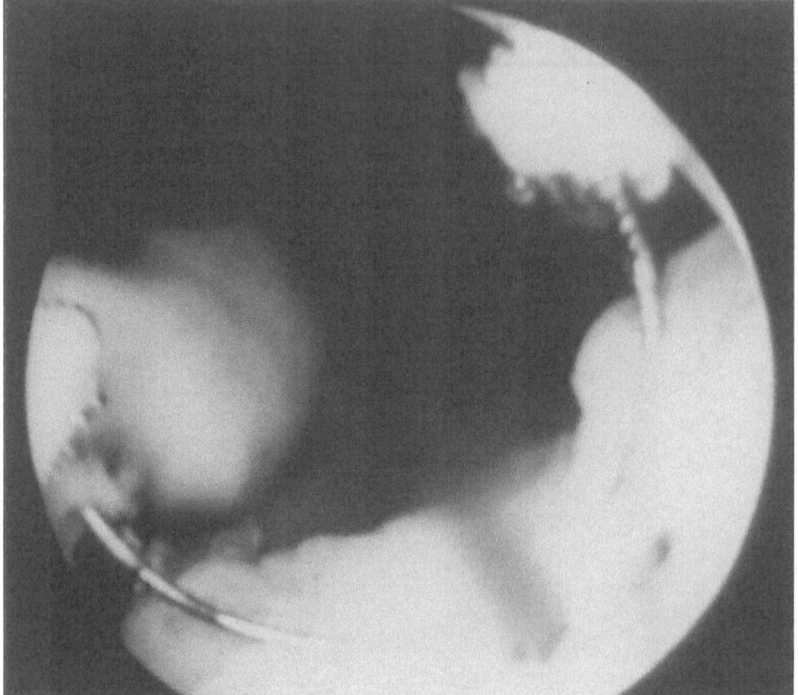

Fig. 5. Magnified video image on the monitor, showing a bleeding vessel

present means that the teacher can intervene much more easily to correct the student. Other staff also become more involved in the operation; the anesthetist, for instance, can see how the operation is progressing and fine-tune the anesthesia correspondingly. Video TUR also, of course, leaves the surgeon open to constant scrutiny and criticism.

Following a short period of training and readjustment an experienced surgeon can perform video TUR using only the monitor for orientation after the first few procedures. The video image is of such high quality and yields such good exposure that the surgeon no longer needs to look through the eyepiece. The magnification (up to 50-fold) renders bleeding points more readily identifiable than with the conventional TUR technique, with the result that hemorrhage is more readily halted. Over the course of the 2 years up to the time of writing, average intraoperative blood loss was reduced by more than 40% (Fig. 5).

An absolute requirement for good video visualization is optimal flow. This is ensured by the use of the continuous-flow resectoscope and, when necessary, preoperative suprapubic paracentesis (Cystofix),

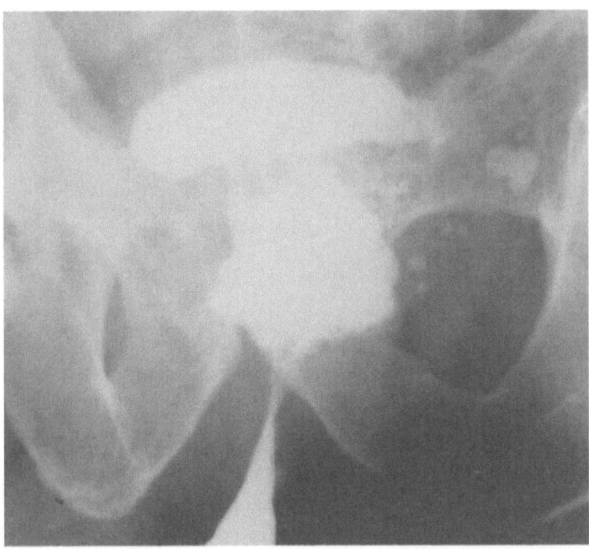

Fig. 6. Urethrocystography after complete clearance of the concavity of the gland and video TUR of an adenoma weighing 55 g

thus avoiding the obscuring of the visual field by blood, the so-called red-outs [17, 24]. If video TUR is performed without a continuous-flow resectoscope, cystostomy is necessary.

Resection by means of video TUR is more convenient than conventional TUR, particularly in cases where the latter requires the surgeon to sit in a contorted position. Even at the roof of the concavity of the gland, between 11 o'clock and 1 o'clock, complete resection and precise hemostasis can be achieved easily and without contortions simply by altering one's grip on the resectoscope.

Somewhat surprisingly, no problems are encountered even with resection at the apex either side of the colliculus; even without direct vision, orientation presents no difficulties. After just a short learning phase periodic checks via the eyepiece are no longer necessary and the resection time drops dramatically.

Excellent detail can be perceived by virtue of binocular vision and the great magnification of the image. The surgeon can thus target the tissue for resection much more effectively and can remove even very small adenomas, particularly at the apex. This complete clearance is demonstrated on urethrocystography (Fig. 6). The result is a marked improvement in flow rate; the majority of our patients exhibit a rate of more than 30 ml/s after video TUR (Fig. 7).

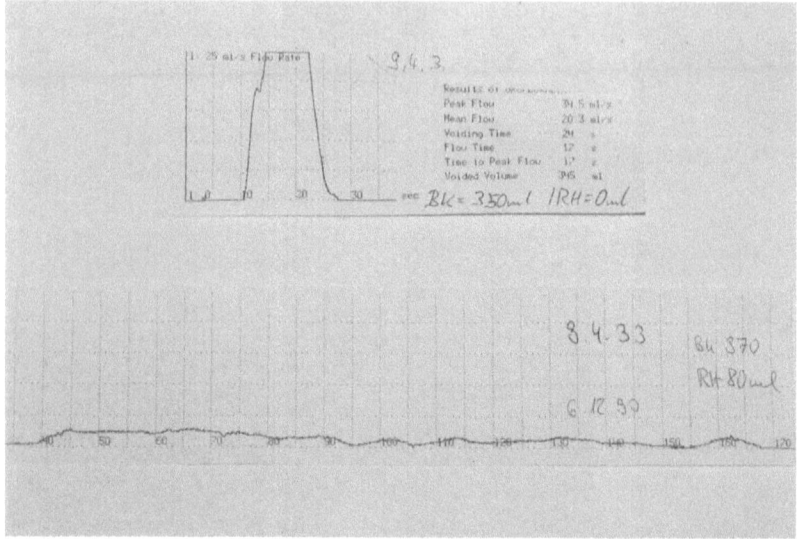

Fig. 7. Flow rates before and after video TUR: postoperative flow rate 30 ml/s

Using the above-mentioned camera and generator, we have never experienced reduction in image quality due to problems with the electricity supply during cutting, and only occasionally during coagulation. Even then the operation has never had to be interrupted.

Video TUR relieves surgeons who wear glasses from the tiresome misting over of the lenses that so frequently occurs on conventional TUR.

The surgeon does have to become accustomed to constantly adjusting the position of the camera (with the left hand) in order to check that the loop is always correctly positioned (Figs. 8–10). The Olympus minichip camera we use is connected to the eyepiece so loosely that the camera always returns to the 6 o'clock position due to its own weight.

The advantages of video TUR as outlined above apply equally to *transurethral resection of bladder tumors*. Adequate orientation is no problem, and the excellent resolution affords accurate assessment of cutting depth and differentiation of structures, enabling radical resection of tumors whose stage permits. Even tumors at the roof of the bladder, like those in a corresponding position in the prostate, can be resected without any concortions on the part of the surgeon as long as the grip on the resectoscope is suitably modified.

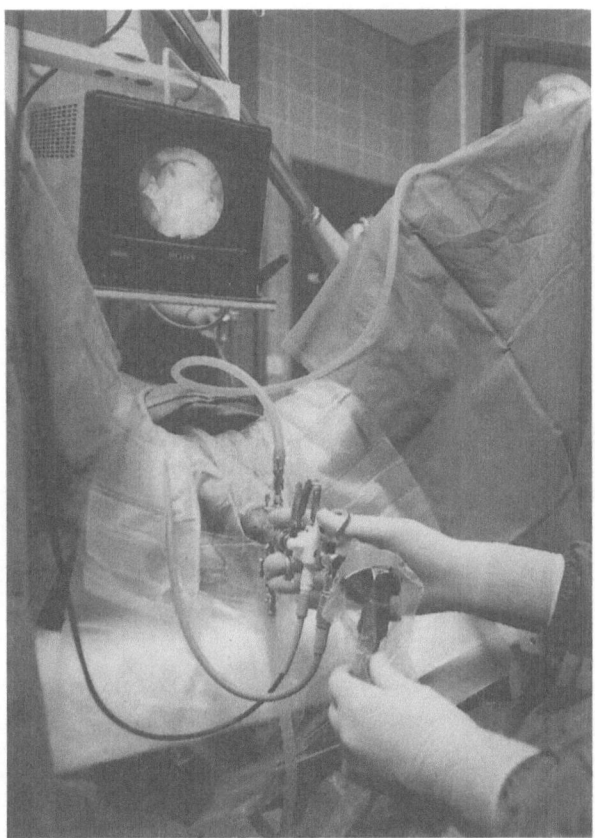

Fig. 8. TUR at 12 o'clock, camera at 6 o'clock: note altered grip with thumb on top (resectoscope rotated 160°)

Advantages and Disadvantages

The advantages and disadvantages of transurethral resection under video guidance can be summed up as follows.

Advantages for the Surgeon and Other Personnel

- The surgeon's comfortable sitting (or standing) position lessens fatigue, decrease the strain on the spinal column („TUR surgeon's syndrome"), and thus reduces long-term damage.

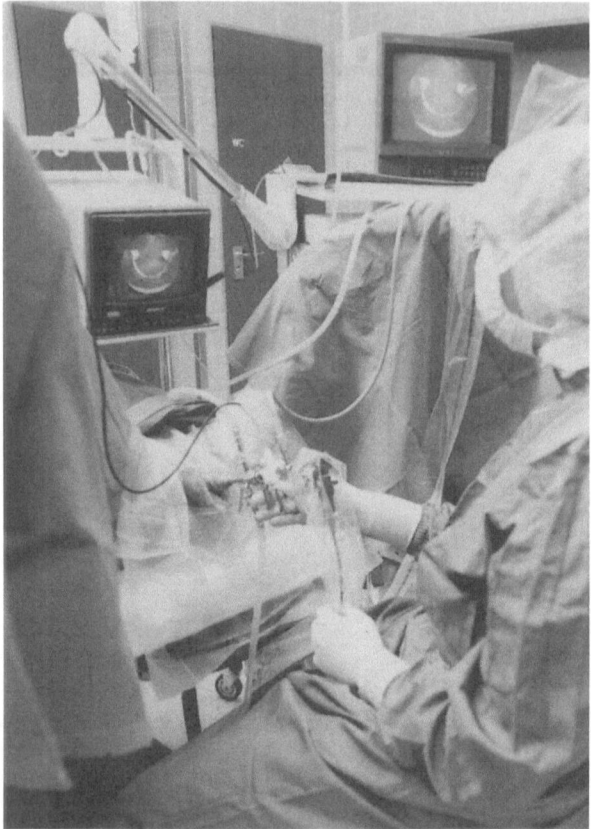

Fig. 9. TUR at 6 o'clock, camera also at 6 o'clock

- The transurethral procedure can be demonstrated more readily and can also be followed by other members of the operating team (e.g., assistant, nursing staff, anesthetist), greatly increasing their interest in the operation.
- In an operation being carried out by a surgeon learning the video technique, the teacher can take over at any appropriate moment. The procedure can also be recorded on video tape for purposes of teaching and discussion.
- Video TUR is still easier to perform than conventional TUR when access is hampered, for instance in a patient with coxarthrosis or a large inguinal hernia.
- Contamination with urine, and thus the risk of infection (AIDS, hepatitis, nonspecific infection, etc.), is greatly reduced.

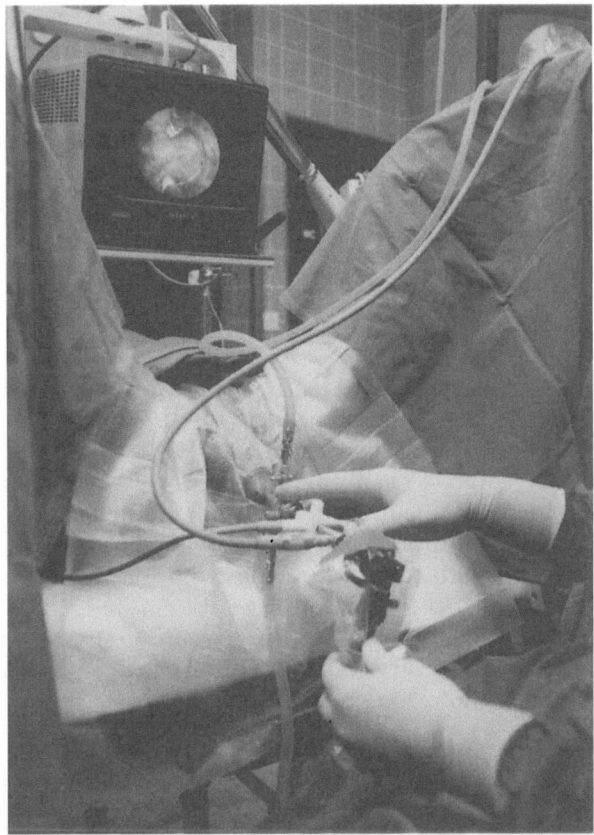

Fig. 10. TUR at 3 o'clock, camera at 6 o'clock

- Surgeons who wear glasses are no longer at a disadvantage.
- The video technique can be extended to all other endourological procedures.

Advantages for the Patient

The advantage of video TUR for the patient is improvement in results.

- The surgeon's binocular vision and the 40- to 50-fold magnification of the image enable more effective hemostasis and thus reduce blood loss.

- The magnification also enables transurethral resection of even the smallest adenomas. Complete resection can be easily and reliably achieved even in ventral and apical locations, resulting in better postoperative flow rates.
- The reduced discomfort for the surgeon and the use of low-pressure irrigation lead to a decrease in resection time.
- The shorter resection time reduces the mechanical trauma to the urethra and thus lowers the stricture rate.

Disadvantages

The disadvantages of video TUR are mostly temporary in nature.

- There is a short learning phase.
- The surgeon has to adjust to possibly unaccustomed equipment, procedures, and conditions, such as the continuous-flow resectoscope, cystostomy, and the 400-W light source.
- A conventional resectoscope can be used only if cystostomy is also performed; optimal flow has to be ensured.
- Rectal digital control of the transurethral resection is hampered by the fact that the left hand is often occupied with adjusting the camera position.

Concluding Remarks

It remains to be seen whether the advent of the video technique of transurethral resection will lead to complete abandonment of previous methods of performing and teaching this procedure, as has already happened in other disciplines, for example in orthopedics with operations on the knee joint. What is already clear, however, is that a new era has dawned in the treatment of benign prostatic hyperplasia. The improved comfort for the surgeon and the better postoperative results of video TUR are raising the gold standard.

References

1. Appleton GVN, O'Boyle PJ, Lumb GN (1984) Video prostatectomy versus conventional TUR. 3rd Congress of Endourology, Karlsruhe, p 324
2. Berner W, Tscherne H (1982) Video-Technik bei der Arthroskopie. Unfallheilkd 85:441−443
3. Davies JH, Harrison GSM (1991) Should urologists wear spectacles for transurethral resection of the prostate? Br J Urol 67:182−183
4. Faul P (1977) Erfahrungen mit dem Dauerspülresektoskop von Winter und Ibe an der Urologischen Abteilung des Stadtkrankenhauses Memmingen. Urologe [B] 17:243−244
5. Faul P (1990) Die Video-TUR. Urologe [A] 29:286−290
6. Faul P, Partecke G (1989) Der autologe Blutersatz in der Urologie. Urologe [A] 28:88−93
7. Geister H (1977) Weitere Erfahrungen mit dem Dauerspülresektoskop „Modell Stade". Urologe [B] 17:242
8. Gillquist J (1980) Operation arthroscopy. Endoscopy 12:281−287
9. Gillquist J, Karpf PM (1982) Arthroskopische Operationen am Knie. Fortschr Med 100:51−55
10. Gioaninni P, Sinocco A, Cariti G (1988) HIV infection acquired by a nurse. Eur J Epidemiol 4:119−120
11. Hartung R, Ley H (1991) The TUR of the prostate. State of the art. J Endourol 5 [Suppl 1]:586
12. Iglesias JJ, Stams UK (1977) Über die Wichtigkeit der kontinuierlichen Absaugung für die hydraulische Haemostase bei der transurethralen Resektion der Prostata. Urologe [B] 17:234−238
13. Jackson RW (1978) Videoarthroscopy: a permanent medical record. Am J Sports Med 6:213−216
14. McNicholas TA, Jones JJ, Sibley GNA (1989) AIDS: the contamination risk in urological surgery. Br J Urol 63:565−568
15. O'Boyle PJ, Lumb GN, Appleton GVN (1984) Videoprostatectomy. Brd Congress of Endourology, Karlsruhe, p 323
16. O'Boyle PJ, Raina S, Holdoway AT (1989) Videoprostatectomy. Guidelines for choosing an effective microvideo operating system. Br J Urol 63:624−626
17. Osawa T (1989) Transurethral resection of the prostate under television monitoring (TV-TUR P). 7th World Congress on Endourology and ESWL, Kyoto
18. Perez Castro E (1977) Erfahrungen mit dem Iglesias-Resektoskop. Urologe [B] 17:238−239
19. Planz C, Chiari R (1977) Transurethrale Elektroresektion mit und ohne kontinuierliche Spülung im Vergleich. Urologe [B] 17:241
20. Rodney WM, Dusanian LL, Werblun MN (1985) Second generation video sigmoidoscopy. Am Fam Phys 31:127
21. Sivak NJ Jr, Fleischer DP (1984) Colonoscopy with a videoendoscope. Preliminary experience. Gastrointest Endosc 30:1
22. Tajima A, Suzuki K, Oktawana Y, Fujita K (1984) Application of the video system in urological endoscopy. Hinyokika Kiyo 30:13
23. Widran J (1985) Videoprostatectomy. Urology 29(2):191−192
24. Widran J (1988) Video transurethral resection using controlled continuous flow resectoscope. Urology 31(5):382−386
25. Yachia D (1987) Videoprostatectomy or armchair prostatectomy. Urology 30:189

Transurethral Resection of the Prostate in Benign Prostatic Hyperplasia

H. Borchers[1] and G. Jakse[2]

Introduction

Transurethral resection of the prostate (TURP) for benign prostatic hyperplasia (BPH) is the most common operation in urology and one of most common operations in medicine in general. In the United States 350000 resections were performed in 1985 [16]. According to Arrighi et al., 0.4% of those aged 55–59 years receive prostatectomy annually. This figure increases to 3.7% in men aged 80–84 years [2].

It is important to consider the treatment of choice in a disease with a very high incidence and which entails enormous costs in Western health systems. Even the United States Congress has shown interest in the treatment of BPH [11, 12]. This chapter on transurethral prostatectomy does not seek to summarize completely the recent discussion about TURP but reviews present indications, techniques, and complications. It is very surprising that so much discussion can be devoted to an operation that is well established and has been performed successfully for decades. Moreover, we should keep in mind that TURP may remain the only adequate and definitive treatment of BPH, and in a few years the present discussion of prostatectomy may have been forgotten completely.

History

In the sixteenth centruy Paré performed the first transurethral procedure on a man with an infravesical obstruction; the patient suffered from an urethral stricture. After this early event advances in endourology were very few. The invention of the electral light by Edison in 1879

---
[1] Kantonsspital Basel, Departement Chirurgie, Spitalstraße, CH-4031, Swizerland
[2] Urologische Klinik, Medizinische Fakultät der RWTH, Pauwelsstraße 30, W-5100 Aachen, FRG

was the first really important step on TURP. The cystoscope was developed independently by Nitze and Leiter in 1887, and 1924 the electrical knife by Waapler and Wyeth followed. In 1932 McCarthy performed the first early form of TURP. Eleven years later Nesbit described a method very similar to the transurethral prostatectomy of today [21] and is considered the „father" of TURP.

Indications

There are many indications for TURP. These may be divided in absolute, relative, and elective ones. The differing views on performing TURP lead to different numbers of resections in countries with otherwise comparable conditions in terms of medical standards. Differences can also be observed in various areas of the same country [29].

Absolute Indications

One absolute indication for TURP acute urinary retention (Table 1). Blandy recommends resection before retention reccurs but not immediately after the event [5]. He reports that resection as a cold case results in up to 10% lower mortality than that directly after acute retention. If there is significant residual urine due to BPH, the prostate must be resected. In these cases the patient presents with symptoms of prostatism and may later develop upper urinary tract obstruction. Today, this in combination with overflow incontinence is seen rarely. Better and earlier medical care spares patients from this serious complication of BPH. Transurethral prostatectomy is required operability has been achieved via urinary diversion by suprapubic or transurethral drainage and conservative treatment.

Another absolute indication for transurethral prostatectomy is recurrent urinary infection due to an infravesical obstruction. Painless

Table 1. Absolute indications for prostactectomy. (From [18])

Significant residual urine	34.4%
Urinary retention, acute	27.1%
Recurrent urinary infection	12.3%
Hematuria	12.0%
Altered urodynamic function	9.9%
Renal insufficiency	4.5%
Bladder stones	3.0%

hematuria may also occur from BPH. In cases of recurrent hematuria it is necessary to resect the prostate. Other causes of hematuria must of course first be excluded. Bladder stones are rare today. These may be caused by BPH or other urological and neurological diseases. If BPH is the cause of these stones, the prostate must be resected and the stone removed. Large bladder stones often require open prostatectomy because the procedure of endourological lithotripsy may last too long.

Relative Indications

Hypertrophy of the detrusor muscle in a early stage is a relative indication for prostatectomy (Table 2). Progression of this process can lead to the development of diverticula and to a hypo- or even atonic bladder. Before irreversible changes in the bladder muscle occur, TURP should be performed; however, the appropriate time cannot be determined.

It is current clinical practice to perform TURP in men presenting with symptoms such as poor stream, hesitancy, and terminal dribbling. Other symptoms of prostatism involve frequency and nocturia. Here the aim of the operation is improvement in the patients quality of life and not the elimination of obstruction, confirmed preoperatively by urodynamics or the evidence of absolute indications. Barry et al. and Fowler et al. [3, 8] pointed out that these patients do not have to be operated on, but that the operation may be performed. Only when the patient is informed about the chances and the risks of prostatectomy, can he make a reasonable decision.

Elective Indication

Enlarged size of the gland itself, for example, as measured by transrectal ultrasound, should not lead to TURP. In urodynamics small adenomas can cause obstruction while large ones do not. Blandy observes that even rectal palpation does not help the surgeon decide

Table 2. Relative indications for prostatectomy. (From [24])

Frequency	61.7%
Nocturia	64.5%
Dysuria	33.1%
Urge	23.2%
Stress incontinence	5.7%
Urge incontinence	5.1%

whether to resect [5]; he sees the value of this standard urological examination only in the discovery of carcinomas of the prostate or large bowel. Thus, if a prostate is large but nonobstructive, and the patient is otherwise well, the indication for prostatectomy is elective. There is a good argument for operating before the patient develops severe problems due to obstruction if he also has other medical problems such as coronary heart disease or diabetes mellitus.

It should be emphasized, however, that the relative and elective indications must be ssen in the light of less invasive treatment alternatives discussed elsewhere in this volume.

Besides the history and clinical examination, the diagnostic examinations needed for deciding whether to perform TURP include ultrasound, uroflow measurement of the residual urine, urography, and urethrocystoscopy. For verification of the suspected obstruction, urodynamic considerations are important. In current clinical practice, however, the examinations routinely performed preoperatively differ from one urologist to the other. Urodynamic examinations, for example, is not generally performed routinely due to lack of staff or facilities or to excessive costs.

Surgical Technique

The procedure of transurethral prostatectomy still follows the principles established by Nesbit in 1943 [21]. Prostatectomy is a step-by-step operation. After having resected the adenoma near the bladder neck, a prominent bladder neck can be incised as described by Turner Warwick. Kulb et al. reported that this prevents postoperative bladder neck contracture [15]. The next step is resection of the lateral lobes. Some surgeons resecting in quadrants while others resect one side after the other. Differing areas for orienting incisions are described. Resection of the area close to the external sphincteric mechanism deserves special attention as the last step of prostatectomy. In cases of inadequate removal of the adenomatous tissue in this area both the immediate and the long-term results may be disappointing.

The existence of a wide variety of techniques, as described by Mebust [16] and Hartung [10], indicates that each offers certain advantages. Resection to the surgical capsule can be attained by all the modifications of the Nesbit technique.

Transurethral incision of the prostate is an interesting variation. Orandi first described this technique in 1973 [22]. He incised the prostate over the total length in 5 and 7 o'clock position with or without continuing bladder neck incision. Orandi considered this approach to be indicated in cases of obstruction without measurable enlargement of the gland. He reported that patients with prostates weighing up to 20 g can be treated in this way, leading to less erectile impotence and retrograde ejaculation, which is important especially in younger patients. The technique is more difficult in larger glands, and the results are unpredictable.

Today, 24-F resectoscopes are used for prostatectomy. Irrigation is intermittent or continuous; as irrigating fluid a nonhemolytic iso-osmotic solution is used. Small-caliber catheters (18–20F) are left in place for 1–2 days postoperatively.

Complications of TURP

Perioperative Complications (Short-Term)

Complications may be urological or nonurological in nature. The most common urological problems are failure to void and intraoperative and postoperative bleeding (Table 3).

Blood loss during prostatectomy is of clinical relevance only when a venous sinus is opened. In a retrospective study in TURP patients Pientka et al. found an average hemoglobin decrease of 2.9 ± 1.6 g/l; in 12.7% of patients the decrease in hemoglobin was 5.0 g/l or more [24]. In 1988 Staehler et al. recommended the intraoperative retransfer of erythrocytes, obtained via cell saver separating blood from cell detritus and irrigation fluid. This normally avoids the transfer of donor blood and diminishes the risk of infection by hepatitis or HIV [27].

Arterial bleeding from uncoagulated arteries results in postoperative clot retention. This bleeding usually leads to a significant blood loss within a very short time. After evacuation of the clot retention, the bleeding can be stopped by further increasing the volume of the balloon. If this strategy fails, the bleeding vessels must be coagulated in a second-look operation. Other complications of TURP include infection of the prostatic fossa, epidydimitis, and septicemia, occurring in 2.3%–5% of cases [18, 28].

Table 3. Perioperative complications. (From [16])

Failure to void	6.5%
Bleeding	3.9%
Clot retention	3.3%
Infection	2.3%

Apart from intraoperative invasion of bacteria and resulting inflammation of the prostatic fossa, perforation of the prostatic capsule and the subsequent contact of urine with the periprostatic tissue may cause long-standing dysuria and fibrosis. To prevent contact between urine and the area of perforation, the indwelling catheter and/or the suprapubic drainage should be removed later then normally.

The occurrence of urosepsis is generally due to urinary tract infections which were insufficiently treated preoperatively. Today, urosepsis due to transurethral prostatectomy is rare, but it is the main cause of operative mortality [18].

Among medical complications, cardiovascular disease is of most clinical relevance in TURP patients; this is particularly so with increased age. Pientka et al. reported that 37% of all resected patients have had a history of cardiovascular disease of some degree. Hypertension and chronic obstructive airways disease are also common in these patients [24]. In combination with extensive blood loss, as described above, and absorption of irrigation fluid, severe complications include myocardial infarction (0.7%), pulmonary embolism (0.3%), and cerebral stroke (0.5%), and these contribute to mortality after TURP [24].

A new method for monitoring intraoperative irrigation fluid absorption has recently been described by Hulten et al. [14]: by adding 1% ethanol to the irrigation fluid, the amount of absorbed fluid is determined by measuring expired ethanol using a breath alcohol analyzer. According to these authors, early detection of absorption and a rapid beginning of therapy decreases the percentage of TUR syndrome (2%) and leads to a reduction in cardiovascular complications after TURP [18]. Further results are presented in a separate chapter of this volume.

Postoperative Complications (Long-Term)

Postoperative dysuria is the principal long-term complication (Table 4). This occurs frequently after prostatectomy and forces the patient who has just undergone surgery for dysuria to return to his physician.

Table 4. Long-term complications (data from various sources)

Reoperation	2.0% – 16.0%
Bladder neck contracture	2.7% – 10.0%
Stricture	2.5%
Incontinence	0.5% – 4.0%
Impotence	4.0% – 40.0%

Table 5. Cumulative probability of undergoing a second prostatectomy, according to geographic location and type of initial prostatectomy (in percent; from [26])

Time after operation	Denmark TURP	Open	Manitoba TURP	Open	Oxford Region TURP	Open
1 year	4.3	1.2	2.3	0.6	3.2	0.8
5 years	9.7	3.4	9.6	2.1	8.9	1.1
8 years	12.0	4.5	15.5	4.2	12.0	1.8

There are various possible courses that postoperative dysuria may take. One must distinguish between dysuria caused by incomplete resection of the adenoma, by bladder neck contracture, and by shrinking of the prostatic capsule. Depending on their degree, these may result in a reoperation. The rate for this has been reported at 2%–16% [4, 5, 7, 20, 25]. This wide range results from differing follow-up times and from differing numbers of patients in the surveys. There are varying views among urologists regarding indications for a second operation, just as regarding those for primary TURP.

In 1989 Roos et al. reported that there is a substantially higher rate of a second operations among patients receiving TURP than in those receiving open prostatectomy (Table 5). This was explained by the more complete removal of prostatic tissue in open operation [26].

In a small series Bruskewitz et al. found bladder neck contracture in about 10% of resected patients; all were patients with small adenomas [6]. However, bladder neck contracture is not uncommon when large adenomas must be treated by open prostatectomy [1]. In other studies, however, such as the cooperative investigation reported by the American Urological Association, the number was much smaller; in only 2.7% was this complication observed [18].

Strictures of the urethra occur in 2.5% of all cases [18]. These are caused either by injuries to the urothelium by the resectoscope or by inflammation and irritation due to postoperative catheterization, despite the use of silicon catheters. For prevention, small-caliber resectoscopes should be used and the catheter removed within 1–2 days.

Urinary incontinence after prostatectomy is a serious complication of TURP. In the series of Fowler et al. incontinence was seen in 4% out of a total of 263 cases at 1 year postoperatively [8]. In the cooperative study, however, only 0.5% suffered from severe incontinence, and another 1.2% showed mild symptoms of stress incontinence [18].

Another risk of prostatectomy, one regarding which the patient must be informed preoperatively, is retrograde ejaculation. This is of importance especially in younger, sexual active men. Between 4% and

40% of patients report either retrograde ejaculation or erectile impotence after TURP [9, 13]. More detailed information about this is presented in a separate chapter of this volume.

Results

The list of early and late complications after TURP suggests that this operation is hazardous and entails unpredictable results. However, this impression is incorrect. Most patients benefit from the operation, overcoming their symptoms and their infravesical obstruction. Modifications based on the expertences of skilled surgeons have made the operation even more efficient. Urologists in the United States reported in a poll that they felt that transurethral prostatectomy must be performed more often than four other major urological operations (TUR of the bladder, suprapubic prostatectomy, ureterolithotomy, and radical cystectomy) before the urologist is experienced in performing it [11].

Morbidity was 18% in the cooperative study and thus represented no change in comparison to previous data [18]. Mortality, however, has decreased over the past 60 years; there has been a gradual reduction from 5% in the 1930s [23] to 2.5% in 1962 [22], 1.3% in 1974 [19], and 0.2% in 1987 and 1989 [18, 25]. In 1987 Roos and Ramsey noted that this figure is age related; in men aged 75 years or older mortality rate is fives as high as in younger men [25]. Motality in the first three of the above studies was caused predominantly by cardiovascular disease – myocardial infarcation and pulmonary embolism – but in the cooperative study urosepsis was the main factor in death after TURP [18].

Roos et al. reported in 1989 that mortality after TURP is higher than after open operations (Table 6). This can be explained by the confounding influence of difference in the preoperative state of health, as urologists seldom offer open prostatectomy to more severely ill patients. However, even in patients who are healthy preoperatively the

Table 6. Cumulative risk of death after surgery according to geographic location and type of operation (in percent; from [26])

Time after operation	Denmark		Manitoba		Oxford Region	
	TURP	Open	TURP	Open	TURP	Open
90 days	2.47	2.67	1.73	1.57	4.39	3.21
1 year	7.55	5.76	5.97	4.18	10.32	7.64
5 years	31.05	25.49	25.37	21.14	35.42	26.45
8 years	46.50	39.78	39.25	33.53	49.49	38.42

Table 7. Success rate after TURP in symptomatic patients (in percent; from [8])

Preoperative symptoms	Symptoms in the year after TURP		
	Better	Same	Worse
Severe	93	7	
Moderate	79	15	6
Mild	80	20	

number of deaths is higher. So far there is no convincing explanation for the association between transurethral prostatectomy and the increased long-term risk of death [26].

Surprisingly few data exist regarding the long-term outcome after prostatectomy. Bruskewitz et al. reported that 1 year after surgery 84% and 3 years postoperatively 75% of patients benefit from the operation [6]. Meyhoff reported that even 5 years after TURP 90% of patients were still satisfied with their results [20]. Fowler et al. divide their series of resected men on the basis of preoperatively determined changes in micturition (Table 7). They found that after 1 year thos with severe symptoms had benefited most from the operation. Only 7% shawed unchanged problems after surgery. Among patients with moderate symptoms there was no improvement in 15% and a worsening in 6%, while 20% of those with mild symptoms perceived no change or worsening after prostatectomy [8].

Thus, patients benefit most from transurethral resection of the prostate when their selection is based on subjective (symptoms) and objective (obstructive) findings. However, even in hands of experienced urologists a certain number of patients will have disappointing results. A thorough urodynamic evaluation may help to decrease the percentage of these patients (W. Schäfer, personal communication).

References

1. Altwein JE, Rüffen H (1991) (1986), Urologie, 3rd Enke Munich
2. Arrighi HM, Guess HA, Metter EJ, Fozard JL (1990) Prostate 16:253
3. Barry MJ, Mulley AG, Fowler FJ, Wennberg JW (1988) Watchful waiting versus immediate transurethral resection for symptomatic prostatism. JAMA 259/20:3010–3017
4. Bergman RT, Turner R, Barnes RW et al. (1955) Comparative analysis of one thousand cases of transurethral prostatectomy. J Urol 74:533
5. Blandy JP (1978) The indications for prostatectomy. Urol Int 33:159–170
6. Bruskewitz RC, Larsen EH, Madsen PO et al. (1986) 3-Year follow-up of urinary symptoms after transurethral resection of the prostate. J Urol 136:613–615

 7. Chilton CP, Morgan RJ, England HR et al. (1978) A critical evaluation of the results of transurethral resection of the prostate. Br J Urol 50:542—546
 8. Fowler FJ, Wennberg JE, Timothy RP, Barry MJ, Mulley AG, Hanley D (1988) Symptom status and quality of life following prostatectomy. JAMA 259/20:3018—3022
 9. Hargreave TB, Stephenson TP (1977) Potency and prostatectomy. Br J Urol 49:683—688
10. Hartung R (1990) Die transurethrale Elektroresektion der Prostata. Akt Urol (Suppl: Operative Techniken) 21:1—10
11. Holtgreve HL (1990) American Urological Association survey of transurethral prostatectomy and the impact of changing medicare reimbursement. Urol Clin North Am 17/3:587—593
12. Holtgreve HL, Valk WL (1962) Factors influencing the mortality and morbidity of transurethral prostatectomy: a study of 2015 cases. J Urol 87:450—459
13. Holtgreve HL, Valk WL (1964) Late results of transurethral prostatectomy. J Urol 92:51—55
14. Hulten JO, Sarma VJ, Hjertberg H, Palmquist B (1991) Monitoring of irrigating fluid absorption during transurethral prostatectom. Anaesthesia 46:349—353
15. Kulb TP, Kamer M, Lingema JE et al. (1984) Prevention of post-prostatectomy vesical-neck contracture by prophylactic vesical-neck incision. J urol 137:277—279
16. Mebust WK (1990) Transurethral prostatectomy. Urol Clin North Am 17/3:575—585
17. Mebust WK, Holtgreve HL, Cockett ATK (1989) Transurethral prostatectomy: immediate and postoperative complications. A cooperative study of 13 participating institutions evaluating 3885 patients. J Urol 141:243—247
18. Melchior J, Valk WL, Foret JD (1974) Transurethral prostatectomy: computerized analysis of 2223 consecutive cases. J Urol 111:640—643
19. Meyhoff HH (1987) Transurethral versus transvesical prostatectomy: clinical, urodynamic, renographic and economic aspects. A randomized study. Scand J Urol Nephrol Suppl 102:1—26
20. Nesbit RM (1943) Transurethral prostatectomy. Thomas, Springfield
21. Orandi A (1990) Transurethral resection versus transurethral incision of the prostate. Urol Clin North Am 17/3:601—612
22. Perrin P, Barnes R, Hadley H et al. (1976) Forty years of transurethral prostatic resections. J Urol 116:757—758
23. Pientka L, van Loghem J, Hahn E, Keil U (1991) Häufigkeit und Komplikationen der Prostataadenomchirurgie bei Patienten mit benigner Prostatahyperplasie. Urologe [B] 31:211—216
24. Roos NP, Ramsey EW (1987) A population-based study of prostatectomy: outcomes associated with differing surgical approaches. J Urol 137:1184—1188
25. Roos NP, Wennberg JE, Malenka MPH, Fisher ES, McPherson K et al. (1989) Mortality and reoperation after open and transurethral resection of the prostate for benign prostatic hyperplasia. N Engl J Med 320:1120—1124
26. Staehler G, Jänicke U, Schmiedt E, Stelzer J (1988) Autologe Re-Transfusion gewaschener Erythrozyten bei der transurethralen Resektion/TUR) von Prostataadenomen. Urologe [A] 27:218—220
27. Symes JM, Hardy DC, Suthern K et al. (1972) Factors reducing the rate of infection after transurethral surgery. Br J Urol 44:582—586
28. Wennberg JE, Mulley AG Jr, Hanley D, Timothy RP, Fowler FJ et al. (1988) An assessment of prostatectomy for benign urinary tract obstruction. JAMA 259:3027—3030

TURP Syndrome:
Monitoring of Immunologic Parameters
and Breath-Ethanol Content
During Transurethral Prostatic Resection

M. Sohn[1], C. Vogt[1], G. Heinen[2], N. Nordmeyer[3], and G. Jakse[1]

Introduction

Recent epidemiological studies [1, 2] have raised serious concerns regarding long-term mortality following transurethral prostatectomy due to myocardial damage. With an increasing spectrum of alternative semi- or noninvasive treatment modalities it is of the utmost importance to evaluate in detail all possible risk factors of this standard procedure in prostatic hyperplasy. The so-called transurethral resection of the prostate (TURP) syndrome, which occurs in 2%−7% of all transurethral prostatic resections, was first described by Creevy four decades ago [3] and consists of an acute toxic fluid overload to the patient's circulation. Since the introduction of isoosmotic irrigation solutions the clinical manifestations have changed from hemolysis with resultant icterus and acute renal failure to individual syndromes ranging from dizziness and confusion to acute systemic circulation breakdown.

Three major pathogenetic components have been seen as responsible for its manifestation: septicemia by circulating endotoxins, sudden blood loss, and sudden intravascular fluid overload [4]. Hyponatremia as a major laboratory finding does not itself produce the clinical manifestations; sudden intravasal hypoosmolality is probably the most significant cause of clinical signs [4]. Severe hyponatremia *without* hypoosmolality remains asymptomatic [5]. Hypoosmolality and hypervolemia secondarily lead to hypovolemia due to low intravascular oncotic pressure with resultant fluid shifts to interstitial spaces [6].

[1] Urologische Klinik, Medizinische Fakultät der RWTH, Pauwelsstraße 30,
W-5100 Aachen, FRG
[2] Abteilung für Immunologie, Medizinische Fakultät der RWTH, Pauwelsstraße 30,
W-5100 Aachen, FRG
[3] Abteilung für Anästhesiologie, Medizinische Fakultät der RWTH,
Pauwelsstraße 30, W-5100 Aachen, FRG

Capillary dysregulation may be even aggravated by circulating endo-toxins, resulting in severe hypotension and bradycardia with impend-ing multiorgan failure. The effect of an acute blood loss in this situation may be deleterious, but it is difficult to quantitate due to the afore-men-tioned simultaneous dilution.

Even without clinical signs of severe fluid absorption hemodynamic evidence of perioperative cardiac stress has been found [7]. This sup-ports the suspicion of long-term morbidity and mortality after trans-urethral prostatic resection [1]. The need for a simple and reliable monitoring parameter for fluid absorption and the uncertainty about the influence of endotoxinemia during transurethral resections were the reasons for starting a prospective interdisciplinary study at our institution.

Material and Methods

A total of 52 consecutive patients entered the study; in 41 of these, parallel immunologic monitoring was possible. The mean age was 68.2 years and mean resection time 48.6 min. Of the 52 patients 46 showed benign prostatic hyperplasia and 6 patients prostatic carcinoma during histologic work-up. The mean weight of resected material was 29.25 g. All patients received parenteral antibiotic prophylaxis; 30 received a single shot of 200 mg ciprofloxacin (Ciprobay, Bayer, FRG). The irri-gation fluid used during resection was Purisole SM (Fresenius, FRG) containing 270 g sorbite and 54 g mannite per 10. Ethylethanol was added to the irrigation fluid, resulting in a 2% concentrated solution. All patients were operated on under spinal anesthesia. No anesthesia-related complications occurred.

Every 5 min patients were requested to inspire deeply and exhale into the mouthpiece of an alcometer device (Alcotest 7110) with inte-grated override function (Dräger, FRG). The system consists of an infrared absorption analysis of the ethanol content of expired breath, including a calculator-assisted program for breath volumes less than 1000 ml („override function"). The system is connected to a keyboard and printer for complete documentation (Fig. 1).

Blood samples were taken every 10 min for laboratory tests includ-ing: ethanol measurement (dehydrogenase assay and gas chromatog-raphy), hemoglobin, sodium, potassium, and urea.

Every 10 min the central venous pressure, heart frequency, systolic and diastolic arterial pressure, body temperature, and state of con-ciousness were recorded. Parallel to hemoglobin controls by our cen-tral laboratory a new pocket-sized photometer test system (HemoCue-

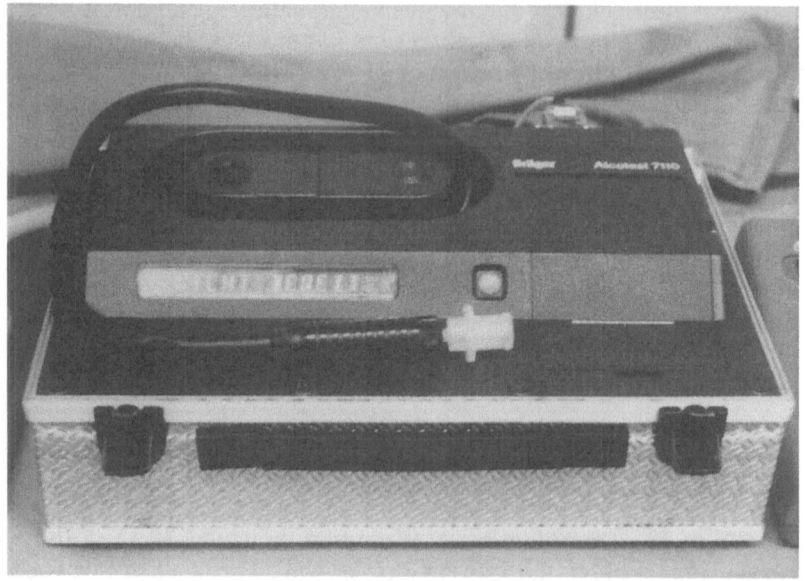

Fig. 1. The Alcotest 7110 (Dräger, FRG) with keyboard and integrated override-function

System, Biotest, FRG) was used for bed-side measurement. The same system was applied for measurement of blood loss from the collected blood-stained irrigation fluid. During resection there was continuous ECG monitoring.

Blood samples were taken before, 30 and 90 min, and 24 h after the start of resection for enzyme-linked immunosorbent assay for tumor necrosis factor (TNF; MABS, Knoll, FRG).

At the same intervals tests were performed for acute-phase proteins such as C-reactive protein, ceruloplasmin, 1-glycoprotein, and haptoglobin as well as two different tests for evidence of circulating endotoxins (LAL-Test, Haemachem, St. Louis, USA; QCL-Test Whitaker-Bioproducts, Walkersville, USA). The study design was approved by the Ethics Committee of the Medical Faculty of RWTH Aachen.

Results

For calculation of absorbed irrigation fluid *(A)*, the Widmark formula was used: $A = C \times P \times R$, where C is ethanol breath content, P is body weight, and R is a sex-dependent resorption and metabolization coefficent.

The mean fluid absorption was 746 ml. Only 11 of the 52 patients did not absorb irrigation fluid during resection. The distribution of absorption volumes in all patients is described in Fig. 2. There was a close correlation between maximum ethanol breath content and maximum ethanol serum ($r = 0.94$). Between the parameters exists a linear correlation (Fig. 3). There was a significant difference between the sodium values before the beginning of fluid absorption and the point of maximum absorption ($p = 0.0001$), while no linear relationship existed to breath ethanol values ($r = 0.39$; Fig. 4). Hemoglobin values differed significantly between the beginning and the maximum point of absorption, but no linear correlation to ethanol breath values was established.

There was no correlation between resection time and fluid absorption ($r = 0.26$) nor between weight of resected tissue and fluid absorption ($r = 0.05$). The median blood loss (calculated from hemoglobin content of collected irrigation fluid) was 0.61. No correlation existed between the amount of blood loss and maximum ethanol breath values ($r = 0.37$). A significant difference was found between central venous pressure at the beginning of the operation and the point of maximum absorption ($p = 0.017$), but no linear relationship was established to corresponding ethanol breath values ($r = 0.65$). Heart-frequency, systolic and diastolic arterial blood pressure and body temperature did not

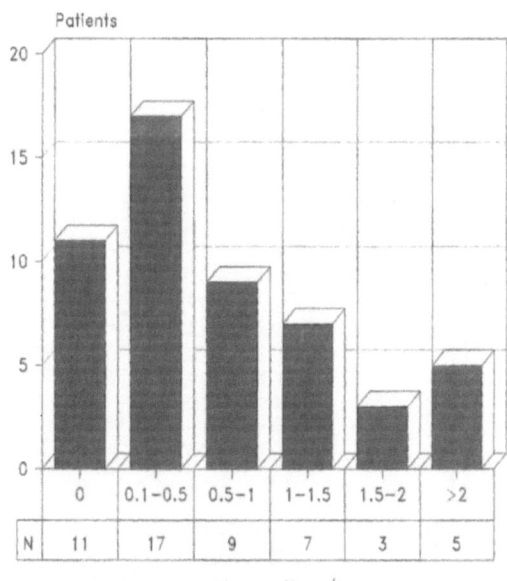

Fig. 2. Distribution of irrigant fluid absorption in all patients ($n = 52$)

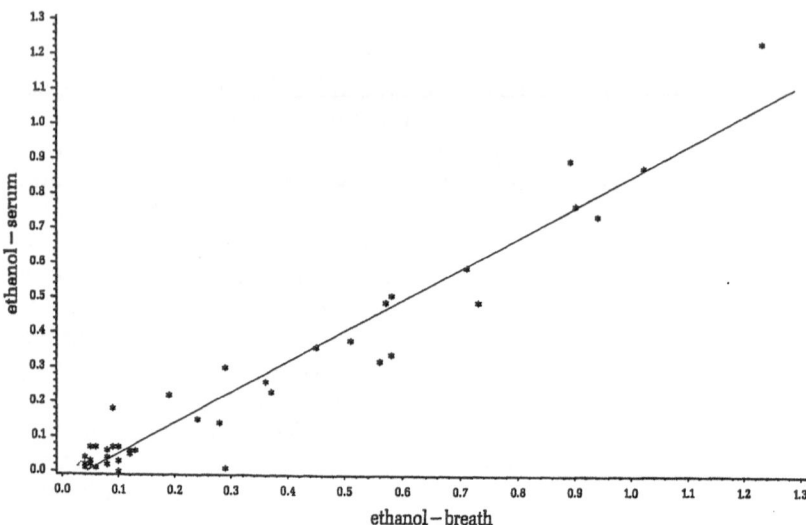

Fig. 3. Correlation between maximum ethanol breath content and maximum ethanol serum content in all patients ($n = 52$)

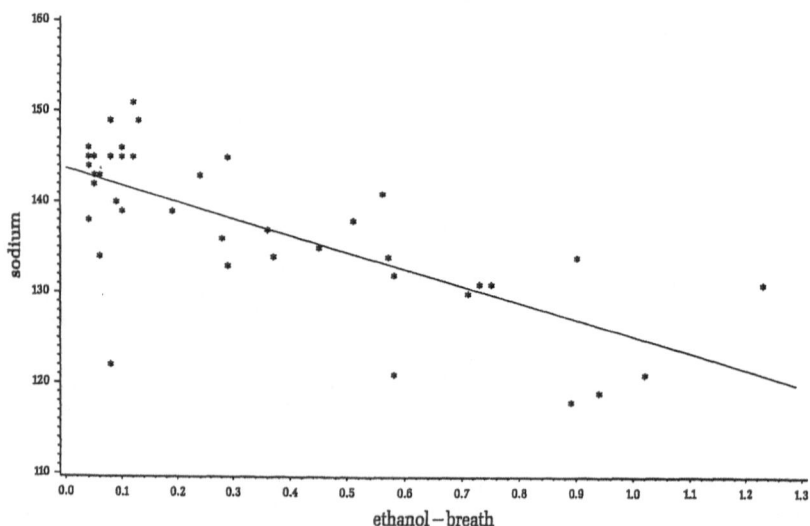

Fig. 4. Correlation between maximum ethanol breath content and sodium values in all patients ($n = 52$)

change in a linear relationship to maximum ethanol breath values, but a significant decrease in heart frequency and rise in diastolic pressure at the point of maximum fluid absorption was found ($p = 0.01$ and 0.029, respectively).

Four patients showed clinical symptoms of a beginning TURP syndrome. Circulating endotoxins were found in 11 of 41 examinations. A preexisting urinary infection was diagnosed in 5 of these 11 patients, but also in 15 endotoxin-negative patients. All patients received parenteral antibiotic prophylaxis before the start of resection. No acute-phase proteins showed any significant rise in correlation with the amount of fluid absorption. A rise in TNF values to $250-1000$ pg/ml (normal < 60 pg/ml) after 60 min of resection was observed in four patients. Three of these four patients showed clinical signs of TURP syndrome. All four patients had positive tests for endotoxinemia at the time of the TNF rise. Two further patients showed constantly high values of TNF (>1000 pg/ml); both had a prostatic carcinoma and showed no clinical or laboratory signs of fluid absorption.

Discussion

Hulten and coworkers were the first to describe the simplicity of estimating fluid absorption during transurethral resections by ethanol breath monitoring [8]. Hahn adopted the idea and verified its high sensitivity and reliability in several studies [9, 10]. The necessity of obtaining breath volumes of more than 1500 ml limited its usefulness in this geriatric population.

The new infrared device presented in this study was developed for forensic purposes (traffic controls, etc.) to avoid serum alcohol measurement. Its reliability has recently been verified according to the recommendations of the Organisation Internationale de Métrologie Légale [11]. The integrated override function permits the evaluation of breath volumes even below 1000 ml. The correlation between ethanol breath and ethanol serum measurement was highly significant ($r = 0.97$; Fig. 3).

In this study a 2% alcohol solution was used as irrigation fluid. It is remarkable that absorption volumes of more than 2000 ml occur without any clinical signs. Of our patients 16% absorbed more than 1.5 l irrigation fluid. Clinical symptoms of TURP syndrome occurred at lower absorption volumes in three out of four patients. On the other hand, endotoxinemia seems to be a frequent event during transurethral prostatic resection. Eleven of 41 patients showed this phenomenon, but only four of these presented acute clinical symptoms. All but one of

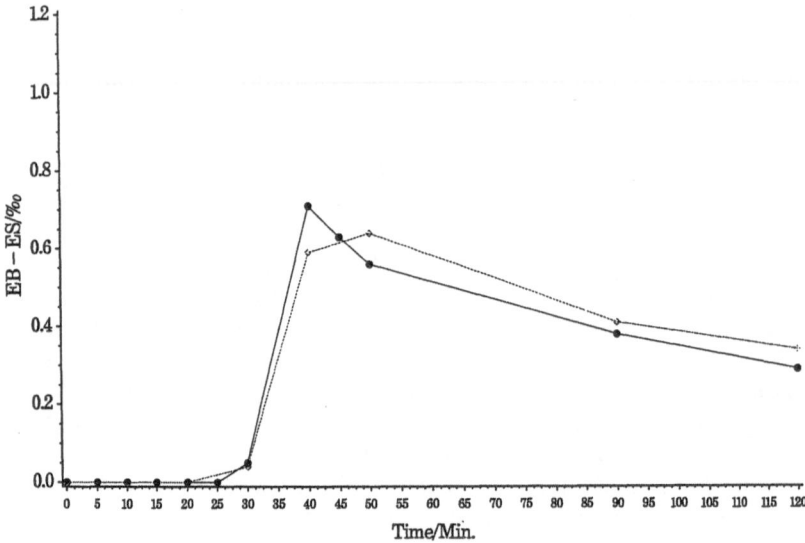

Fig. 5. Fast fluid absorption after inadvertent opening of periprostatic veins: sudden rise of ethanol breath content; ●————● ethanol breath, ◇– – –◇ ethanol serum

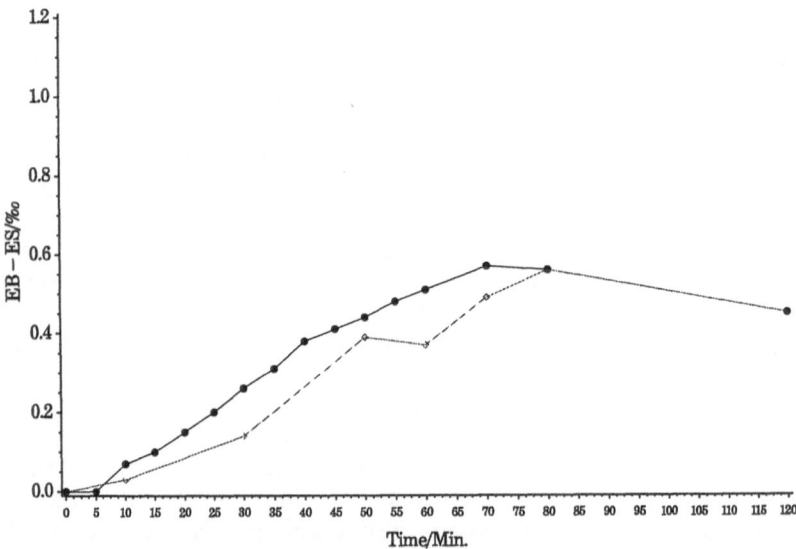

Fig. 6. Slow but continuous fluid absorption during resections of large adenomas. During resection, alcohol metabolism takes place and reduces blood and breath ethanol content; ●————● ethanol breath, ◇– – –◇ ethanol serum

these four patients showed substantial rise in TNF, which seems to be an indicator of threatening sepsis. It is also impressive that routine preoperative screening for urinary infection and routine intraoperative antibiotic coverage does not prevent septic reactions during transurethral resections.

Ethanol breath monitoring permits a highly reliable intraoperative supervision of transurethral resections. It is superior in sensitivity and cost effectiveness to all other reported methods of absorption monitoring. Nevertheless, two pitfalls should be mentioned. The Widmark formula has been developed for the purpose of calculating slow alcohol uptake by the gastrointestinal tract. Thus an equal distribtuion of alcohol is presumed in all body fluid compartments. This is not the case if alcohol enters the lung circulation by direct intravenous application, such as in massive absorption through periprostatic veins. In this case the ethanol breath content reflects the *intravascular,* not the *intracorporeal* alcohol content (Fig. 5), which leads to an overestimation of absorbed irrigation fluid.

On the other hand, prolonged continuous absorption, as may occur during resection of large adenomas, underestimates the true intravascular fluid uptake due to parallel alcohol metabolism, which is between 0.1 and 0.2‰ per hour (Fig. 6).

With these limitations in mind, ethanol breath content measuring with the Alcotest 7110 remains a cheap, highly reliable monitoring method.

Recently, Evans and coworkers demonstrated in a small but well-designed study that transurethral resections even without any clinical or laboratory signs of fluid absorption lead to an important increase in myocardial work and oxygen demand due to increased left ventricular afterload [7]. This may be deleterious for geriatric patients with compensated but severely compromised cardiopulmonary reserves. They may survive the operation without any evidence of cardiovascular decompensation, but their condition declines comparable to that after a survived myocardial infarction. In this context the influence of endotoxin induced liberation of TNF may increase the myocardial malnutrition due to microvascular coagulation and endothelial damage.

If these results are confirmed in further studies, the role of transurethral prostatectomy must be questioned in the light of emerging alternatives and more conservative treatment modalities.

References

1. Roos N, Wenneburg JE, Fisher ES (1989) Mortality and reoperation after open and transurethral resection of the prostate for benign prostatic hyperplasia. N Engl J Med 320:1120−1124
2. Wenneburg JE, Roos N, Sola L (1987) Use of claims data systems to evaluate health care outcomes mortality and re-operation after prostatectomy. JAMA 257:933−936
3. Creevy CD (1956) Hemolysis and transurethral resection. Surgery 39:180−188
4. Ghanem AN, Ward JP (1990) Osmotic and metabolic sequelae of volumetric overload in relation to the TUR-syndrome. Br J Urol 66:71−78
5. Wright HK, Gann DS (1962) Severe postoperative hyponatraemia without symptoms of water intoxication. Surg Gynecol Obstet:553−556
6. Guyton AC, Coleman TG (1968) Regulation of interstitial fluid volume and pressure. Ann N Y Acad Sci 150:537−547
7. Evans JWH, Suiger M, Chapple CR et al. (1991) Haemodynamic evidence for per-operative cardial stress during transurethral prostatectomy. Br J Urol 67:376−380
8. Hulten JO, Lennart SJ, Wictorsson JM (1986) Monitoring fluid absorption during TUR-P by marking the irrigating solution with ethanol. Scand J Urol Nephrol 20:245−251
9. Hahn RG (1988) Ethanol monitoring of irrigating fluid absorption in transurethral prostatic surgery. Anesthesiology 68:867−873
10. Hahn RG (1989) Early detection of the TUR-syndrome by marking the irrigating fluid with 1% ethanol. Acta Anaesthesiol Scand 33:146−151
11. Schoknecht G, Fleck K, Kophamel B (1989) Die Zuverlässigkeit von Atemalkoholmeßgeräten. Blutalkohol 26:71−86

Urodynamic Assessment in Patients Undergoing Transurethral Resection of the Prostate: A Prospective Study

P.-H. Langen, W. Schäfer, and G. Jakse[1]

Introduction

In the past few years transurethral resection of the prostate (TURP) has gained increasing attention for many reasons. First, there has been the development of alternative methods such as balloon dilatation, hyperthermia, and thermotherapy. Secondly, a growing number of studies provide new data about the effects and efficacy of TURP. In addition, the treatment of benign prostatic hyperplasia (BPH) claims up to a one-quarter of the daily patient care workload of American urologists. And finally, approximately 400000 annually performed transurethral prostatectomies are affecting the costs of public health service and insurance significantly, being responsible for a total of almost $ 4000000000 per year in the United States [11, 13, 14]. Despite the routine that every urologist has in the management of BPH the incidence of TURP varies extremely. This may be due to different criteria in evaluating the need for surgical treatment and different findings about the postoperative outcome [4, 5, 8, 10, 17, 19, 20, 22, 31]. Recently, several studies have reported disturbing postoperative outcomes. Cytron et al. and others found a considerable rate of impotence following TURP [9], and the studies of Roos et al. and Malenka et al. discovered that men undergoing TURP have a higher mortality rate than those in the unoperated surveillance group and a 1.45 : 1 risk of death compared to patients after open prostatectomy [21, 24]. This emphasizes the importance of a standardized objective evaluation of obstruction in order to compare treatments. The indication for surgery is normally based on a variety of subjective and objective parameters [30]. The major ones are

- flow rate and residual urine,
- „irritative“ and „obstructive“ symptoms

---
[1] Urologische Klinik, Medizinische Fakultät der RWTH, Pauwelsstraße 30, W-5100 Aachen, FRG

- morphology (rectal examination, sonography, UCG, cystoscopy), and
- urodynamics (pressure/flow study)

Unfortunately, morphological changes and symptoms of BPH are only loosely connected to any definition of infravesical obstruction [1, 3, 6], but asked about the indication for TURP, the most common answer from urologists will probably be „elimination of infravesical obstruction". The evidence of obstruction is generally furnished indirectly by collecting simple noninvasive data such as flow rate and residual urine. But we must keep in mind that these parameters give only a hint of obstruction. Direct confirmation is given by a pressure/flow relationship as ascertained by urodynamic investigation. Therefore it should be presumed that pressure/flow studies are part of the routine work up prior to surgery. However, this is not the case. A partial reason for this may be the lack of a precise definition of the word „obstruction" or even a quantification (grading) that is commonly accepted [7, 12, 18, 27, 28].

Material and Method

At our clinic we recently conducted a prospective study to determine by urodynamic means whether all patients undergoing TURP are obstructed. A total of 43 consecutive patients referred to our clinic for TURP underwent at least two suprapubic pressure/flow studies both pre- and 1 week postoperatively. All patients were operated on regardless of urodynamic results. The data collected on each patient also included uroflowmetry and postvoiding residual urine measurements from two to six times, confirmation of negative urine culture, and a symptom score based on that used by Jensen et al. [16]. The maximum score was 10 points each for obstructive and for irritative symptoms. The postoperative symptom score was determined by the patients approximately 6 months after surgery. Nine patients did not respond but were included in the analysis of their completed pressure/flow studies. Patients with carcinoma of the prostate and neurogenic bladder disorders were excluded from the study.

Evaluation of Pressure/Flow Studies

We used a new pressure/flow diagram for grading of obstruction, based on the findings on the bladder outlet published by Schäfer [25, 26, 29] and the definition of the passive urethral resistance relation (PURR),

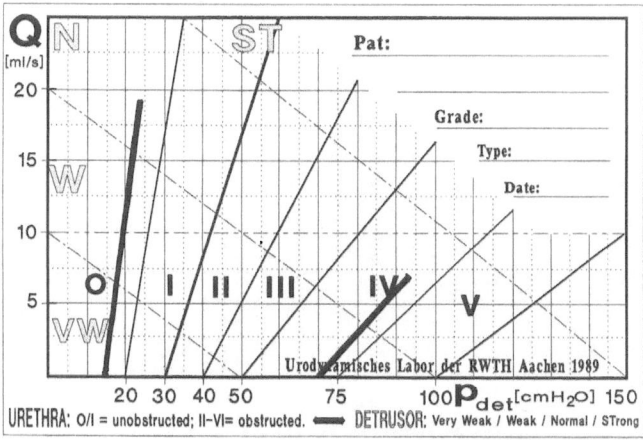

Fig. 1. Diagram for evaluating obstruction caused by BPH

which describes the pressure/flow relation at the flow controlling zone of the bladder outlet independently of detrusor conditions. This distinguishes seven grades of obstruction from nonobstructed to severely obstructed and four grades of detrusor strength from very weak to strong. The classification of each patient can be done in a simple and reliable manner by transferring only two pressure/flow data to the diagram and connecting them by a straight line. These characteristic data points are the pressure at maximum flow and that at minimum flow (minimum urethral opening pressure, p_{muo}). This gives a simplified PURR curve which provides all relevant information that could otherwise be achieved only by computer-assisted analysis of the pressure/flow study (Fig. 1).

The reliability of this method has been confirmed by comparison with computer analysis of more than 1000 pressure/flow studies. Detailed explanation of the diagram is given in another chapter of this volume.

In contrast to urethral strictures, BPH is characterized by compressive obstruction, and p_{muo} is the most important value to characterize it. Ideally, p_{muo} should have identical values at the starting and stopping of flow. However, urodynamic recordings normally show a higher p_{muo} at the start than at the stop of flow, which can be explained by the time delay of the flow recording compared to the recording of the detrusor pressure. Therefore, one must correct the recordings at least roughly for the time delay of one's own urodynamic equipment to determine the correct p_{muo}.

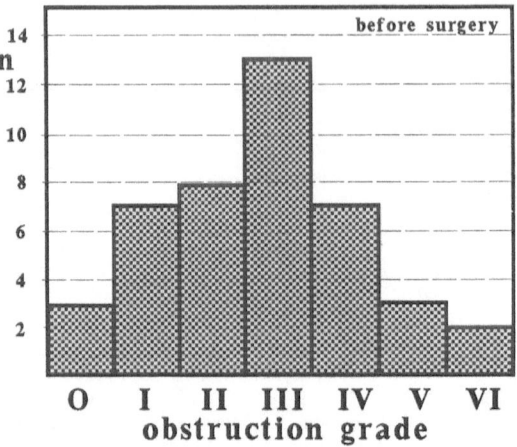

Fig. 2. Preoperative grade of obstruction in 43 patients grouped according to the diagram shown in Fig. 1

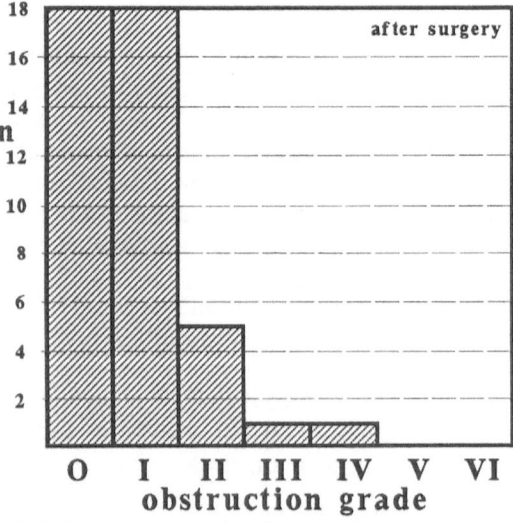

Fig. 3. Postoperative results of 43 patients assessed by urodynamics

Results

Analysis of the data show that TURP is obviously an effective method of eliminating infravesical obstruction. Of our patients 83.6% were in the nonobstructed groups postoperatively. However, there was a remarkably high number of (23%) preoperatively nonobstructed patients (Figs. 2, 3). Does this mean that almost one quarter of the

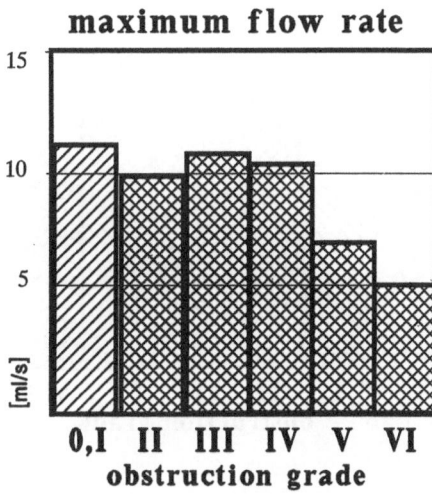

Fig. 4. Comparison of preoperative maximum flow rate and obstruction grade in 43 patient scheduled for TURP

patients underwent unnecessary surgery? Can we identify different characteristics in the obstructed and nonobstructed groups?

Flow Rate and Residual Urine. As already mentioned, obstruction is most commonly investigated by flow rate and residual urine. The −2 standard deviation value for maximum flow rate is 13.5 ml/s, according to Siroky's nomogram. Preoperatively, all patients were below this value. Thus by using flow rate alone infravesical obstruction would also have been assumed in the group of nonobstructed patients (Fig. 4). Regarding residual urine there was no significant difference between the two groups (Fig. 5). These findings explain why an indication for TURP was given for all patients in the eyes of the referring physician. At the same time, they show that flow rate and residual alone are not suitable parameters to confirm obstruction [1, 11, 16].

Irritative and Obstructive Symptoms. As mentioned above, in a quantitative analysis of patients' obstructive and irritative symptoms, the nonobstructed patients showed the higher preoperative scores for obstructive and for irritative symptoms (Fig. 6). The difference was even more impressive postoperatively. In the nonobstructed group the reduction in obstructive symptoms was only 58% while in the obstructed group it reached 76%. The irritative symptom score showed similar changes, with a decline in irritative symptoms of only 61% for nonobstructed patients but 92% for obstructed patients (Fig. 7).

residual urine volume

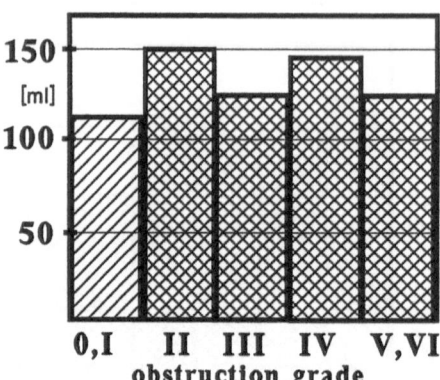

Fig. 5. Comparison of preoperative residual urine volume and obstruction grade in 43 patients scheduled for TURP

pre-operative symptoms

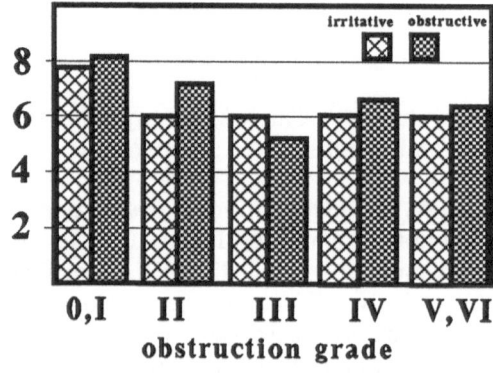

Fig. 6. Comparison of preoperative symptoms and obstruction grade in 43 patients scheduled for TURP

post-operative symptoms

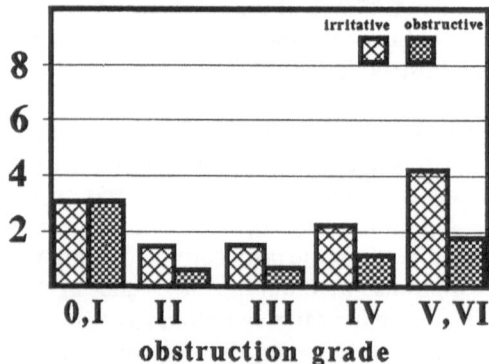

Fig. 7. Comparison of post-operative symptoms and obstruction grade in 43 patients who underwent TURP

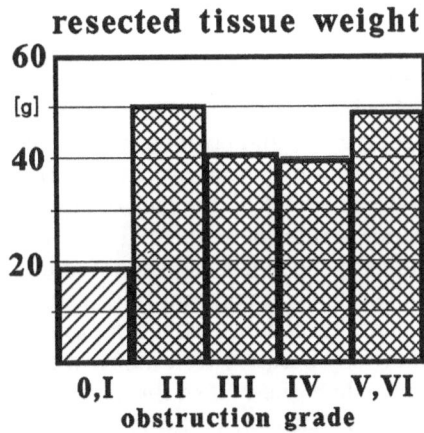

Fig. 8. Comparison of resected tissue weight and obstruction grade in 43 patients

Morphology. Instead of comparing the prostate volumes of the two groups we analyzed the resected tissue weights. We recorded significantly lower weights in the nonobstructed groups (Fig. 8). The mean value for the resected weights of nonobstructing prostates was about one-half that of obstructing prostates (21.5 versus 41.3 g). This may be another hint that the poor voiding function in the urodynamically confirmed nonobstructed groups (0, I) is not caused by BPH but by poor detrusor function.

Pressure/Flow Studies. Evaluation of the urodynamic data by using the new diagram elucidates the accumulation of patients in the obstructed groups II and III (Fig. 2); almost one half of patients (48.6%) presented with mild to moderate obstruction. Postoperatively, 83.6% were in the nonobstructed groups 0 and I. Only two patients remained in group III or IV with moderate obstruction, and no patient was severely obstructed (Fig. 3). While the comparison of pre- and postoperative values for p_{muo} showed no significant changes for nonobstructed patients, all patients defined as obstructed had a significant reduction in p_{muo} ($p < 0.05$). The same was observed for the pressure at peak flow. Only eight patients remained urodynamically unchanged, i.e., within the same group pre- and postoperatively. Except for one they were all nonobstructed patients. Fourteen obstructed patients (42.4%) were classified as having a weak or very weak detrusor, while six out of the ten nonobstructed patients (60%) were found in these classes.

Discussion

Comparison of the different parameters shows that some are of limited value in the decision for surgical treatment [3, 6, 11, 16, 18], such as uroflow rate and postvoiding residual urine volumes. Furthermore, no significant differences between obstructed and nonobstructed patients were observed. In the lack of appropriate data there seems to be a tendency to refer patients for TURP because of symptoms alone, as is indicated by the highest symptom scores for nonobstructed patients.

The low maximum flow rate in nonobstructed patients, which besides their substantial symptoms was another reason for their selection for operative treatment, was found to be a detrusor problem in more than one-half of the cases. However, the meaning of a high rate of weak detrusors in the obstructed group of patients also needs further investigations. A considerably high rate (23%) of patients do not benefit from TURP by urodynamic means. In our study the cutoff point for p_{muo} to define obstruction was 30 cm H_2O. This is even 10 cm H_2O less than suggested by Abrams and Griffiths [3].

The data set from our study is still too small and the follow-up period of 12 months too short to provide definite answers regarding the possible benefits of obstruction grading. Nevertheless, preliminary results from parallel studies unpublished so far using the same grading system show almost identical figures. Up to now more than 100 patients have been included with a follow-up of 6 months or more. Jensen recently reported a satisfaction rate of 85%−90% after surgical treatment of BPH [17]. In our study the overall satisfaction of patients was higher than 90% among obstructed and unobstructed patients. This may be another example of the well-known placebo effects of any treatment for BPH, since no objective changes detectable with full urodynamic investigation have been achieved in the unobstructed group. In spite of this the higher postoperative symptom score in unobstructed patients indicates more unfavorable postoperative outcomes in this group. Therefore, grading of outflow obstruction enables the urologist to include the patient in the decision process for surgical treatment and to be more precise in answering patients' question about the postoperative outcome.

Conclusions

As long as urodynamic investigations with pressure/flow studies are not included in the routine of indication for prostate surgery we must accept that there is a significant number of our patients who may not benefit from the operation. Flow rate alone has a sensitivity in detecting voiding dysfunction of up to 100% (see Fig. 4) but a poor specifity for obstruction of only 70%−80% (77% in our study). Preoperative pressure/flow studies should therefore be accepted as the gold standard for confirming infravesical obstruction. Exact definitions must be elaborated to classify the patients. This could enable us to predetermine the postoperative outcome and to identify the groups that must be treated otherwise (e.g., anticholinergics, thermotherapy, 5α-reductase inhibitors, α-blockers).

Future studies aiming at efficiency or comparison of these treatment modalities should include pressure/flow studies and obstruction grading so that statements such as the following are not longer necessary in the future: „Since well defined criteria that define the minimum symptomatology necessary for surgical treatment simply do not exist, the number of potential candidates for transurethral resection of the prostate is limited to some extent only by the size of the population" [11].

References

1. Abrams PH (1977) Prostatism and prostatectomy: the value of urine flow rate measurement in the preoperative assessment for operation. J Urol 117:70−71
2. Abrams PH, Feneley RCL (1978) The significance of the symptoms associated with bladder outflow obstruction. Urol Int 33:171
3. Abrams PH, Griffiths DJ (1979) The assessment of prostatic obstruction from urodynamic measurements and from residual urine. Br J Urol 51:129−134
4. Abrams PH (1980) Investigations of prostatectomy problems. Urology 15:209−212
5. Abrams PH (1983) Urodynamic results of surgery. In: Hinman F Jr (ed) Benign prostatic hypertrophy. Springer, Berlin Heidelberg New York, p 948
6. Andersen JT, Nordling J, Walter S (1979) Prostatism. The correlation between symptoms, cystometric and urodynamic findings. Scand J Urol Nephrol 13:229−236
7. Andersen JT, Abrams P, Blaivas JG, Stanton SL (International Continence Society, Committee on Standardisation of Terminology) (1988) The standardisation of terminology of lower urinary tract function. Scand J Urol Nephrol Suppl 114, p 7
8. Barry MJ, Mulley AG, Fowler FJ, Wennberg JW (1988) Watchful waiting vs immediate transurethral resection for symptomatic prostatism. JAMA 259:3010−3017
9. Cytron S, Simon D, Segenreich E et al. (1987) Changes in the sexual behavior of couples after prostatectomy. Eur Urol 13:35−38
10. Fowler FJ, Wennberg JE, Timothy RP, Barry MJ, Mulley AG, Hanley D (1988) Symptom status and quality of life following prostatectomy. JAMA 259:3018−3022

11. Graverson PH, Gasser TC, Wassoon JH, Hinman F Jr, Bruskewitz RC (1989) Controversies about indications for transurethral resection of the prostate. J Urol 141:475–481
12. Griffiths DJ (1977) Urodynamic assessment of bladder function. Br J Urol 49:29–36
13. Holtgrewe HL, Mebust WK, Dowd JB et al. (1989) Transurethral prostatectomy: practice aspects of the dominant operation in American urology. J Urol 141:248–253
14. Holtgrewe HL (1991) Outcome research and BPH, new concepts for deciding therapy. American Urological Association update series, vol X, Houston Texas
15. Jensen KME, Bruskewitz RC (1983) Significance of prostatic weight in prostatism. Urol Int 38:173 ff
16. Jensen KME, Jorgensen JB, Mogensen P (1988) Urodynamics in prostatism. Prognostic value of pressure-flow study combined with stop-flow test. Scand J Urol Nephrol Suppl 114:72–77
17. Jensen KME, Andersen JT (1990) Urodynamic implications of benign prostatic hyperplasia. Urologe [A] 29:1–4
18. Khan Z, Mieza M, Bhola A, Starer P (1988) Diagnosis and grading of outflow obstruction. Urology 32:72–77
19. Lepor H, Rigaud G (1990) The efficacy of transurethral resection of the prostate in men with moderate symptoms of prostatism. J Urol 143:533–537
20. McLoughlin KP, Abel PD (1990) Symptoms versus flow rate versus urodynamics in the selection of patients in prostatectomy. Br J Urol 66:303
21. Malenka DJ, Roos N, Fisher ES et al. (1990) Further study of the mortality following transurethral prostatectomy: a chart based analysis. J Urol 144:224–228
22. Meyhoff HH, Gleason DM, Bottaccini MR (1989) The effects of transurethral resection on the urodynamics of prostatism. J Urol 142:785
23. Meyhoff HH, Ingemann L (1981) Accuracy in preoperative estimation of prostatic size. Scand J Urol Nephrol 15:45
24. Roos NP, Wennberg JE et al. (1989) Mortality and reoperations after open and transurethral resection of the prostate for benign prostatic hyperplasia. N Engl J Med 320:1120–1127
25. Schäfer W (1983) Detrusor as the energy source of micturition. In: Hinman F Jr (ed) Benign prostatic hypertrophy. Springer, Berlin Heidelberg New York, pp 450–469
26. Schäfer W (1983) The contribution of the bladder outlet to the relation between pressure and flow rate during micturition. In: Hinman F Jr (ed) Benign prostatic hypertrophy. Springer, Berlin Heidelberg New York, pp 470–496
27. Schäfer W (1985) Urethral resistance? Urodynamic concepts of physiological and pathological bladder outlet function during voiding. Neurourol Urodynam 4:161–201
28. Schäfer W, Ruebben H, Noppeney R, Deutz FJ (1988) Obstructed and unobstructed prostatic obstruction. World J Urol 6:490–497
29. Schäfer W (1990) Principles and clinical application of advanced urodynamic analysis of voiding function. Urol Clin North Am 17:553
30. Walsh A, Marberger H, Morales PA, Murnaghan GF (1983) Indications for prostatectomy – mandatory and optional. In: Hinman F Jr (ed) Benign prostatic hypertrophy. Springer, Berlin Heidelberg New York, pp 771–775
31. Wennberg JE et al. (1988) An assessment of prostatectomy for benign urinary tract obstruction: geographic variations and the evaluation of medical care outcomes. JAMA 259:3027–3030

Erectile Dysfunction
After Transurethral Prostatectomy

R. Sikora, S. Dahms, R. Bosshardt, M. Sohn and G. Jakse[1]

New diagnostic methods such as bidirectional Doppler investigation of penile arteries [1] and intracavernous injections of vasoactive drugs [24] have permitted the quantification of erectile disturbances. Based on sophisticated diagnostic algorithms, various forms of therapy such as intravernous autoinjections of vasoactive drugs [24], revascularization of penile arteries [18], and implantation of penile prosthesis [6] can be offered to the patients.

Anatomy and Physiology of Penile Erection

The penis consists of two corpora cavernosa which communicate with each other through an incomplete septum and the corpus spongiosum covering the urethra. Skin, tunica dartos, and Buck's fascia cover the penile structures. The corpora cavernosa are covered by the rigid tunica albuginea. The basis of the penis is fixed at the symphysis and the abdominal wall by ischiocavernosal and bulbospongiosal muscles [10].

The vascular system of corpora cavernosa is primarily supplied by paired deep penile arteries with corkscrew arterioles. The glans penis is fed by the dorsal penile arteries. These arteries originate from the penile artery, which arises from the internal pudendal artery [9, 13]; (Fig. 1). The venous blood flows from the corpora cavernosa through the venae emissariae, venae circumflexae, and the deep dorsal penile vein into the internal pudendal vein [20a] (Fig. 2).

Pelvic and genital organs are supplied by sympathetic and parasympathetic nerves of the autonomic nervous system. The sympathetic fibers originate from the thoracolumbal segments $T_{10}-L_2$. These run to the presacral area and build the plexus hypogastricus superior. The

[1] Urologische Klinik, Medizinische Fakultät der RWTH, Pauwelsstraße 30, W-5100 Aachen, FRG

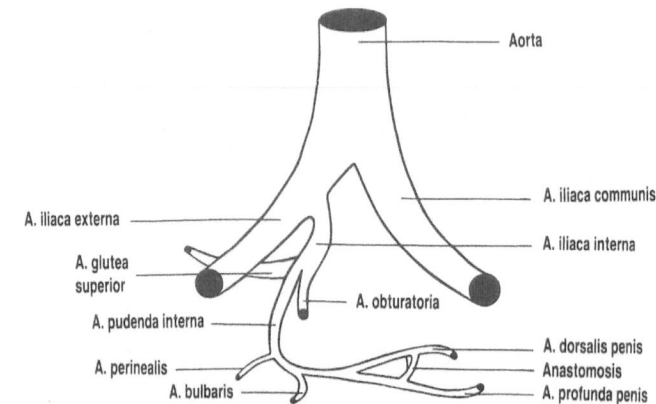

Fig. 1. Arterial supply in the human penis

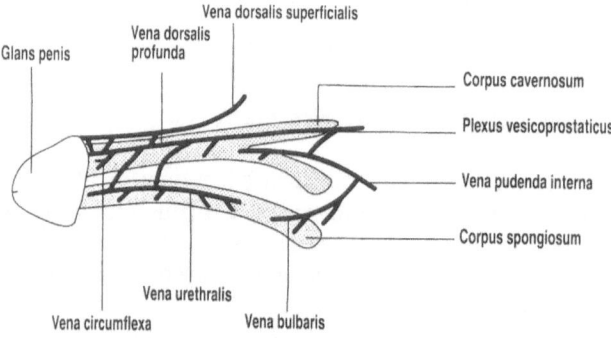

parasympthetic fibers leave the spinal cord by the roots S_2-S_4. They reach the plexus hypogastricus as nervi erigentes, the former containing branches of both autonomic nervous systems [20].

Prostate, seminal vesicle and penis receive their mixed autonomous innervation from the pelvic plexus (plexus hypogastricus inferior) through the plexus prostaticus, the fibers of which run as nervi cavernosi with vessels to the corpora cavernosa after having passed through the diaphragma urogenitale.

Musculus bulbospongiosus and musculus ischiocavernosus are somatomotorically supplied by the pudendal nerve. Topographically these nerves and vessels are closely related to the prostate capsule (Fig.

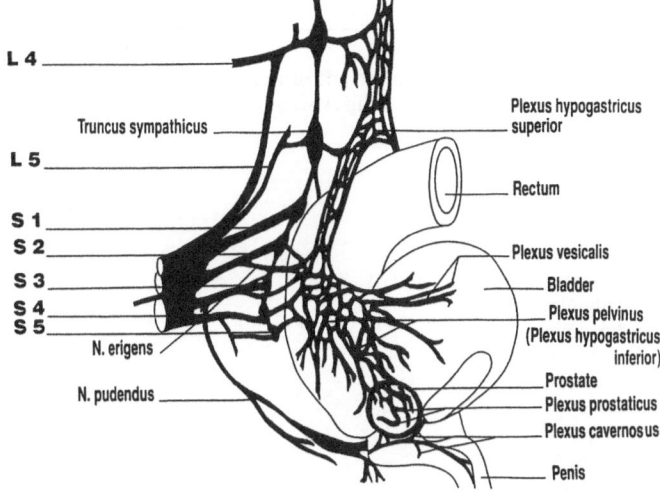

Fig. 3. Innervation of the male genital system

3). In this position, which corresponds to 5 and 7 o'clock, the distance between the apex of the prostate and proximal pars prostatica is 1.5–3 mm [2, 12].

Incidence of Erectile Dysfunction After Transurethral Prostatectomy

Postoperative complications after transurethral resection of the prostate (TURP) in patients with benign prostate hyperplasia (BPH), are well known (Table 1; [3]). However, statements regarding the incidence of erectile disturbances show great variability. According to the literature, the incidence varies between 0% and 40% (Table 2). Penile erection is a complex phenomenon which requires healthy neurological, arterial, venous and psychological conditions. Little attention has so far been paid to evaluating impotence after TURP, which until now has generally been explained by psychogenic factors [15]. In most cases postoperative impotence after TURP has been evaluated by interviews considering the patient's subjective statements. According to these investigations, 69% of those aged 50–70 year [5] and 55% of those 60–80 years old [8] are sexually active. The rate of postoperative erectile dysfunction is 0%–40% [8, 16].

Table 1. Complications of TURP ($n = 1057$). (From [3])

Intraoperative	
Perforation needing exploration and drainage	0.4%
Secondary haemorrhage needing evacuation	2.1%
Pulmonary infection	4.0%
Pulmonary embolism	0.1%
Stroke	0.6%
Coronary thrombosis	0.3%
Postoperative	
Urine culture infected	30.7%
Epididymitis	0.5%
Septicaemia	1.9%
Incontinent	0.5%
Slight symptoms	1.4%
Stricture	
Temporary	1.0%
Permanent	1.3%
Revision	
Within first 3 months	2.1%
4–12 months	3.0%
1–10 years	–

When the patient is informed before TURP about possible post-operative disturbances, the rate of impotence is said to decrease from 63% to 0% compared to those who have not been advised [25].

If, however, objective parameters of nocturnal tumescence measurements are taken into account, the quality of erectile function shows a deterioration of 61.5% in patients after TURP [16]. A correlation between subjective and objective parameters was not found. An additional report shows that 69% of postoperative impotence is due to neurological factors [11]. These authors demonstrated lesions of the pudendal nerve and delayed latent periods of the bulbus cavernosus reflex (BCR).

The comparison between „minimal" and „total" TURP showed no correlation between the postoperative rate of impotence and surgical techniques [19].

Mechanisms of Erectile Dysfunction After Transurethral Prostatectomy

Owing to the close topographic vicinity of nerves and vascular system with the prostate capsule, thermal damage of the cavernosal nerves,

Table 2. Sexual potency before and after TURP by BPH

Reference	Age (mean)	No. of patients	Potent Pre-operatively	Post-operatively
Holtgreve and Valk (1964) [8]	69	840	382	229/382 (60%)
Finkle and Prian (1966) [5]	50–70	102	68	57/68 (83.8%)
Madorsky et al. (1976) [16]	66	14	12	12/12 (0%)
Hargreawe and Stephenson (1977) [7]	64,5	61	61	57/61 (93.4%)
Möller-Nielson et al. (1985) [19]	67	81	58	40/58 (69%)
Bruskewitz et al. (1986) [2a]	ND	69	69	46/69 (66.6%)
Cytron et al. (1987) [4]	ND	90	21	14/21 (66.6%)
Malon et al. (1988) [17]	61.3	58	58	36/58 (62%)
Surya et al. (1989) [22]	69.3	20	20	14/20 (70%)
Keuler und Altwein (1990) [11]	ND	189	189	152/189 (80.4%)

ND: No data available.

thrombosis of the deep dorsal artery, and fibrosis of the corpora cavernosa during and after TURP seems to be possible and makes iatrogenic
erectile dysfunction likely [15]. Perforation of the prostate capsule can
result in a prejudice of the cavernosal nerve due to the formation of
hematoma or of consecutive fibrosis [12]. Most patients who undergo
transurethral prostatectomy are 61–70 years old (Fig. 4), and this age
group presents the highest incidence of erectile dysfunction in the general population. They frequently suffer additional diseases such as
diabetes mellitus or arteriosclerosis [14]. Moreover, they may already
have an unstable balance of neurovascular functions.

Slight operative disturbances such as change in arterial inflow or
venous outflow may result in temporary or permanent erectile dysfunc-

Age

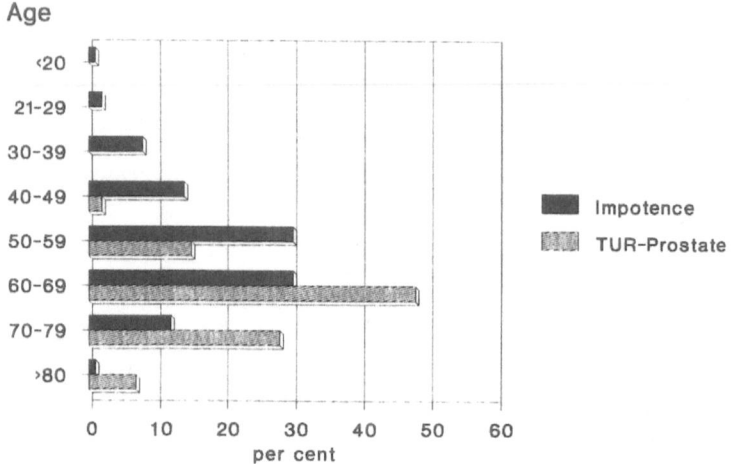

Fig. 4. Age distribution of patients at TUR-P ($n = 1057$) and impotence ($n = 472$). (From [3, 14])

tions [15]. Especially in cases of longer hospital stay, postoperative complications or prostatic cancer, depressions, and anxiety states in older persons additionally impair erectile function [25].

At present, iatrogenic impotence after TURP cannot be excluded. Prospective randomized studies taking into account new diagnostic methods may reveal evidence of an organically caused impotence due to TURP [13, 21, 23].

References

1. Abelson D (1975) Diagnostic value of the penile pulse and blood pressure: a Doppler study of impotence in diabetics. J Urol 113:636−638
2. Breza J, Sherif RA, Brandley RO, Lue TF, Tanago EA (1989) Detailed anatomy of penile neurovascular structures: surgical significance. J Urol 141:437−443
2a. Bruskewitz RC, Larsen EH, Madsen PO, Dorflinger T (1986) 3-Year follow-up symptoms after transurethral resection of the prostate. J Urol 136(3):613−615
3. Chilton CP, Morgan RJ, England HR, Paris AMI, Blandy JP (1978) A critical evaluation of the results of transurethral resection of the prostate. Br J Urol 50:542−546
4. Cytron S, Simon D, Segenreich E, Leib Z, Servadio C (1987) Changes in the sexual behavior of couples after prostatectomy. Eur Urol 13:35−38
5. Finkle AL, Prian DV (1966) Sexual potency in elderly men before and after prostatectomy. JAMA 196:125−129

6. Furlow WL (1979) Inflatable penile prosthesis: Mayo clinic experience with 175 patients. Urology 13:166
7. Hargreave TB, Stephenson TP (1977) Potency and prostatectomy. Br J Urol 49:683−688
8. Holtgrewe HL, Valk WL (1964) Late results of transurethral prostatectomy. J Urol 92:51−55
9. Jünemann K-P, Lue TF, Melchior H (1987) Die Physiologie der penilen Erektion. Urologe [A] 26:283−288
10. Jünemann K-P (1989) Anatomische Voraussetzungen zum physiologischen Ablauf der Erektion. Urologe [A] 28:238−240
11. Keuler F-U, Altwein JE (1990) Ist vor einer transurethralen oder offenen Prostataadenektomie über erektile Impotenz aufzuklären? Urologe [A] 26:A99
12. Lue TF, Zeineh SJ, Schmidt RA, Tanagho EA (1984) Neuroanatomy of penile erection: Its relevance to iatrogenic impotence. J Urol 131:273−279
13. Lue TF, Tanagho EA (1987) Physiology of erection and pharmacological management of impotence. J Urol 137:829−836
14. Lue TF, Müller SC, Jünemann K-P, Fournier GR Jr, Tanagho EA (1987) Hämodynamische Veränderungen während der Erektion und funktionelle klinische Diagnostik der penilen Gefäße mittels Ultraschall und gepulstem Doppler. Akt Urol 18:115−123
15. Lue TF (1990) Impotence after prostatectomy. Urol Clin North Am 17:613−620
16. Madorsky ML, Ashamalla MG, Schussler I, Lyons HR, Miller GH (1976) Postprostatectomy impotence. J Urol 115:401−403
17. Malone PR, Cook A, Edmonson R, Gill MW, Shearer RJ (1988) Prostatectomy: patients perception and long-term follow-up. Br J Urol 61:234−238
18. Michal V, Kramer R, Hejhal L (1973) Direct arterial anastomosis to the cavernous body in the treatment of erectile impotence. Rozhl Chir 52:587−592
19. Möller-Nielsen C, Lundhus E, Moller-Madsen B, Norgaard JP, Simonsen OH, Hansen SL, Birkler N (1985) Sexual life following „minimal" and „total" transurethral prostatic resection. Urol Int 40:3−4
20. Netter FH (1987) Farbatlanten der Medizin. Thieme, Stuttgart
20a. Puech-Leao, Chao S (1988) Venous drainage of the crura − an anatomic study. Proceedings of the 6th Biennial International Symposium for Corpus Cavernosum Revascularisation and 3rd Biennal World Meeting on Impotence. Boston
21. Sohn M, Sikora R, Deutz F-J, Bohndorf K, Günther R (1988) Differenzierte mikrochirurgische Therapie bei vaskulär bedingter erektiler Impotenz. Urologe [A] 27:164−172
22. Surya BV, Macaluso E, Johanson K-E, Brown J (1989) Sexual dysfunction following transurethral resection of the prostate (TUR-P). J Urol 141:220A
23. Virag R, Frydman D, Legman M, Virag H (1984) Intracavernous injections of papaverin as a diagnostic and therapeutic method in erectile failure. Angiology 35:79−87
24. Virag R et al. (1982) Intracavernous injection of papaverine for erectile failure. Lancet 2:938−940
25. Zohar J, Meiraz D, Maoz B, Durst N (1976) Factors influencing sexual activity after prostatectomy: a prospective study. J Urol 116:332−334

Nonoperative Treatment

Are Metallic Endourological Stents an Alternative to Prostatectomy in the Management of Benign Prostatic Hyperplasia?

C. R. Chapple[1]

Introduction

The prostate gland plays an important role in reproductive physiology and commonly undergoes enlargement due to benign hyperplasia (BPH) in elderly men. This occurs with a reported prevalence of 37%−40% during the fifth decade rising to 75%−84% during the eighth decade of life [1, 2]. Indeed, it has been suggested that the chance of a 40-year-old man having a prostatectomy during his lifetime is 29% [3].

Surgical prostatectomy is the traditional therapy of choice for symptomatic BPH. Currently, approximately 90% of patients undergo a transurethral prostatectomy (TURP) [4], and therefore it represents the gold standard, against which other therapies need to be judged. However, in the light of recent work both the efficacy and the safety of prostatic surgery has been questioned [5−12], and this coupled with increased public awareness of alternative non-surgical or minimally invasive treatment options has raised a number of questions as to the appropriate therapy in contemporary practice.

The various froms of therapy include the following:

Conventional surgical prostatectomy
  Transurethral surgery
  Open surgery

Drug therapy
  Alpha-blockade (to relax prostate)
  Hormonal therapy (to shrink prostate)

[1] The Royal Hallamshire Hospital, Department of Urology, Glossop Road, Sheffield S10 2JF, UK

New therapeutic techniques
   Balloon dilatation of the prostatic urethra
   Hyperthermia of the prostate using microwave generators
   Laser therapy
   Ultrasonic cavitation/mechanical pulverisation of the prostate
   Extracorporeal shock wave therapy prostatic stenting

Prostate Stents

This discussion is particularly relevant in the context of the management of the elderly unfit patient, where there has been considerable
interest in the development of a variety of recently developed urethral
devices for stenting and thereby mechanically holding open the prostatic urethra and reducing outflow resistance from the bladder. Of the
many treatments available for treating prostate obstruction, only stents
relieve it to the same degree as surgery. These devices are either temporary or permanent. The principal difference between the two is that
the former are intra-luminal and encrust with phosphatic debris if left
long enough in contact with urine and are liable to become infected.
The permanent stents are more expensive and are under investigation
as a minimally invasive alternative to conventional surgical prostatectomy.

Temporary Stents

Fabian in 1980 [13] first described the use of a „urological spiral" to
relieve urinary retention in two patients. This device consists of a
closely coiled spiral of stainless steel wire narrowed at its inner end to
allow introduction into the urethra and with a single wire at its other
end terminating as a smaller spiral and acting as a tail to facilitate the
adjustment of the position of the stent and allow its easy removal
(Fig. 1). The stent is available in varying lengths. Although this device
works well as a temporary measure [14], it is not without its associated
problems, namely incontinence, urethral strictures, encrustation and
displacement [15]. The stent is easy to insert and remove de novo but
has the disadvantage of any intraluminal appliance in that it is not possible to cystoscope the patient when it is in situ and can be difficult to
remove when encrusted. In an attempt to reduce the potential morbidity associated with encrustation, a gold-plated variant of this stent
which is less reactive has been developed (the Prostakath). Good result
have been reported using this device in patients with acute urinary

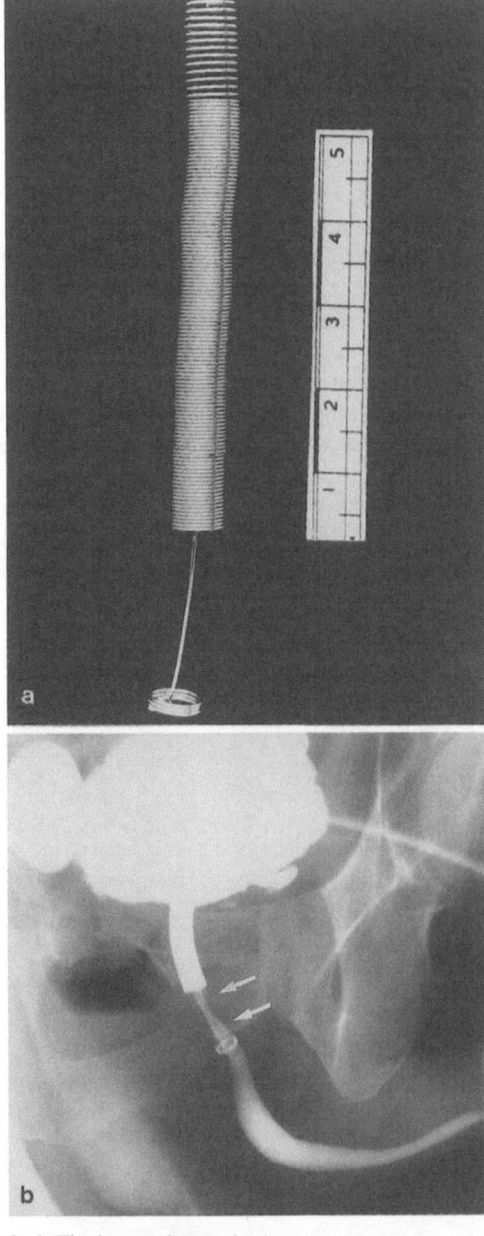

Fig. 1. a The Fabian urological spiral. The long coil rests in the prostatic urethra, the tail lies through the distal sphincter mechanism, and the lower coil helps fix the stent and prevent migration and facilitates removal. **b** The stent in position. *Arrows,* position of the distal sphincter mechanism

retention [16, 17]. The gold plating, however, only delays the inevitable onset of encrustation, and it remains no more than a temporary solution. This stent is easy to insert under local anaesthetic [18] mounted on an introducer and positioned under ultrasound/radiological guidance or under direct endoscopic control. Spontaneous fracture of these stents has been reported [19]. We have occasionally found that during the removal of these devices the wire comprising the fabric of the stent has a tendency to unravel.

The most recent development of this stent has been the use of an alloy with a temperature-dependent shape memory effects, the Memokath. The girth of the base of this stent expands when flushed with 45°C water which helps prevent stent migration.

A new intra-urethral stent constructed of polyurethane and made in variable lengths (45, 55 and 60 mm) with Malecot wings at either end, has been described by Nissenkorn [20, 21] (Fig. 2). The wings are

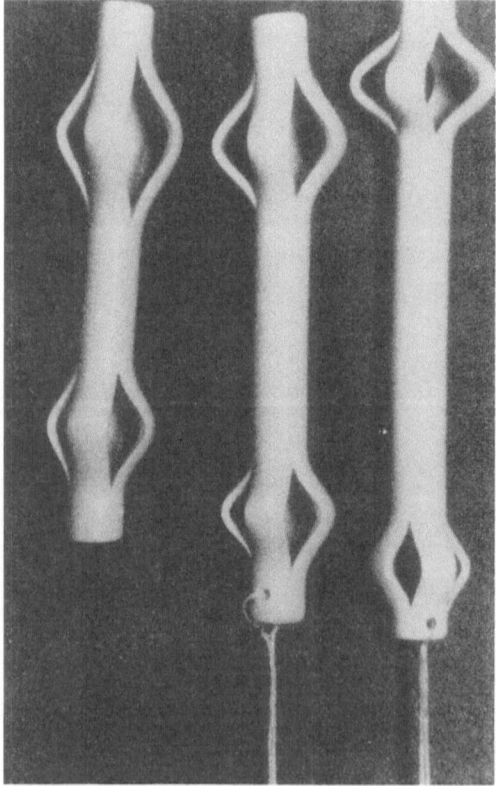

Fig. 2. The Nissenkorn stent

positioned at or proximal to the bladder neck and distal to the verum-ontanum to provide some anchorage and prevent displacement. The appropriate size of stent is chosen after endoscopic measurement of the length of the prostatic urethra, and it is easily inserted with the aid of a purpose built introducer. The stent is supplied with a nylon tail attached to its distal end which facilitates its subsequent removal.

All of these devices provide a temporary solution to the problem of urinary retention in the elderly unfit patient. Certainly, in those patients with a very limited life expectancy, this may provide adequate definitive treatment. The ease of insertion and removal is an advantage in situations where the stent can be regarded as part of the diagnostic process — a form of reversible prostatectomy — for example, in those patients where the relative contributions of a neurological deficit and prostatic enlargement to bladder outflow obstruction are unknown.

Permanent Stents

Two permanently implanted intra-prostatic urethral stents are currently available commercially, the American Medical Systems (AMS) Urolume/Wallstent and the Advanced Surgical Intervention (ASI) titanium stent; alternative devices are under investigation, such as the Gianturco stent [22]. The principal advantage of these stents is that they become completely covered by urothelium and are not intra-luminal. This avoids the complications described above that occur with intra-luminal devices. On theoretical grounds the use of these stents should be the most effective of the current alternatives to the mechanical removal of prostatic tissue. Therefore, although their use has to date been largely confined to the elderly unfit patient, another feature which distinguishes them from the temporary stents is the possibility of using them routinely as a minimally invasive alternative to prostatectomy in the otherwise fit patient.

The ASI Titanium Stent

Stent Insertion

The ASI titanium stent is introduced into the patient loaded in a collapsed state on a modified prostate balloon dilatation catheter (Fig. 3). The correct length of stent is chosen after measurement of the prostate length; the manufacturers recommend endoscopic assessment using a specifically designed calibrated catheter. After introduction and posi-

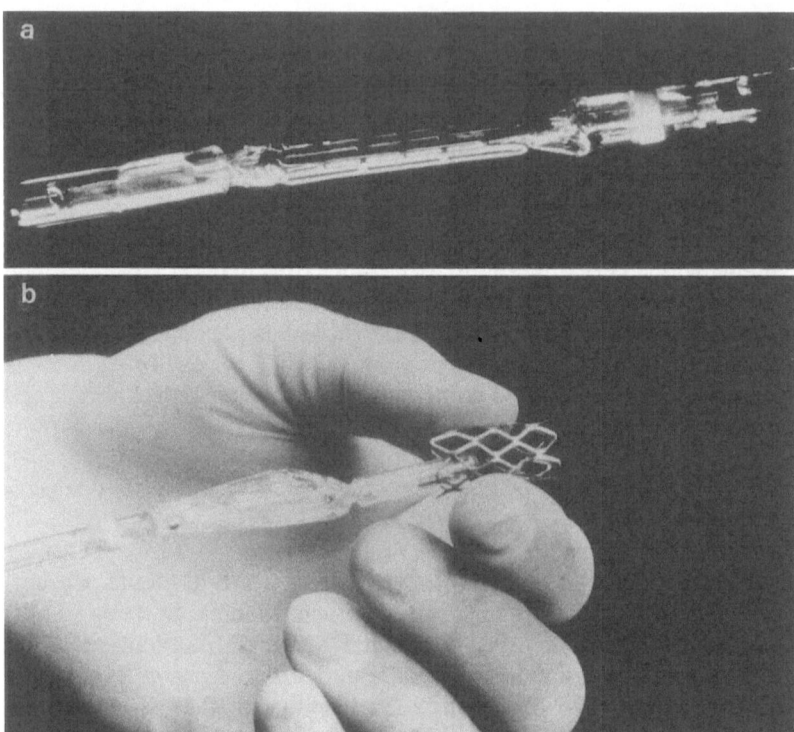

Fig. 3a, b. The ASI titanium stent shown before **(a)** and following **(b)** inflation of the balloon introducer

tioning in the prostatic urethra under endoscopic control, the 12-mm balloon is inflated to approximately 33 F expanding the stent within the lumen. The catheter can then be removed. Although designed for permanant implantation, the stent can be removed endoscopically. The stent is of rigid construction, the cross-sectional area of the frame being greater than that of the fine wire used for the Wallstent.

Results

Initial reports using this device in a total of 64 high-risk patients followed up for a mean of 6 months (1–18 months) have found it to be a satisfactory alternative to prostatectomy, with no evidence of encrustation or significant complications, although asymptomatic bacteriuria was common [23, 24]. Further long-term follow-up of this device is necessary to ascertain how well it covers with urothelium, and whether it remains free from complications. This is particularly relevant in the light of a recent in vitro study investigating the rate of stent encrustation, which suggested it to be more pronounced with this device compared to the Wallstent — possibly related to the greater cross-sectional diameter of the ASI wires and rougher surface as visualised under scanning electron microscopy [25].

The AMS Superalloy Stent

The AMS Urolume stent is a woven tubular mesh of fine grade corrosion resistant nickel superalloy wire manufactured in various lengths and diameters (Fig. 4). It was originally developed for endovascular use and has been used for a number of years in the prevention of stenoses after transluminal angioplasty [26, 27]. Following initial experimental work carried out partly in our unit [28, 29], we have used this stent successfully in the treatment of urethral structures. More recent studies report encouraging results following its use in the prostatic urethra [30, 31].

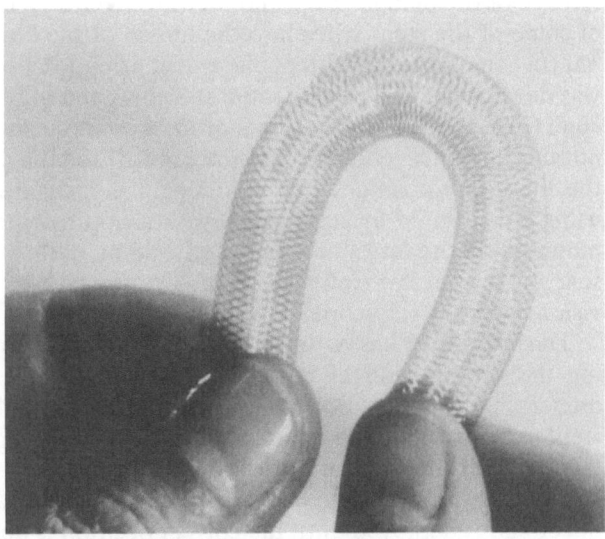

Fig. 4. The AMS Wallstent/Urolume endoprosthesis

Stent Insertion

The original delivery system was a modification of that used for endovascular use. The stent is positioned on a 9-F catheter, held in a compressed and elongated form under a doubled-over plastic membrane. When the space between both layers of the membrane is pressurised to 3 atm with normal saline, the outer layer can be withdrawn allowing the stent to expand within the prostatic urethra. When expanded from its delivery system, the stent is stable though flexible (Fig. 4). The patient lies in the left lateral position. The prostatic urethral length is measured using a linear array transrectal ultrasound (TRUS) and synchronous cystoscopy which identifies the position of the distal sphincter mechanism. The stent introducer is inserted into the bladder over a guide wire. The final deployment of the stent can then be controlled under TRUS guidance. The outer membrane of the stent is peeled back to open approximately one-third of the stent and the whole device gently withdrawn until the proximal end of the opened stent lies at the bladder neck. Once positioned at the bladder neck the stent can be fully opened. In some patients the stent fails to expand fully from its introducer and a 14-mm diameter balloon catheter is passed over the guide wire and inflated within the stent lumen.

Although the catheter-mounted technique allowed positioning of the stent satisfactorily in relationship to the distal sphincter mechanism, it was difficult accurately to delineate the entire circumference of the bladder neck and thereby avoid a significant protrusion of some of the stent wires into the lumen of the bladder. In order to improve the accuracy of stent placement an endoscopic delivery system was developed. The new introducer is designed to be used as a cystoscope (Fig. 5). General, regional or local anaesthesia with urethral lignocaine and intravenous sedation are given, and the patient is placed in the lithotomy position. Prostatic length is measured endoscopically using a calibrated ureteric catheter. An appropriate sized stent premounted on the introducer and sterilised by the manufacturer is chosen, and the device is introduced into the prostatic urethra under direct vision using a 0° telescope.

The introducer has two safety locks. The first is removed after entering the urethra and allows partial stent deployment. Longitudinal movement of the telescope within the device allows the position of the stent to be checked; landmarks such as the verumontanum and the distal sphincter mechanism are visualised through slots cut in the outer sheath (Fig. 6). The stent can be repeatedly pulled back into the introducer and redeployed until the correct position is achieved. Once the final position of the stent is confirmed, ideally covering the entire pros-

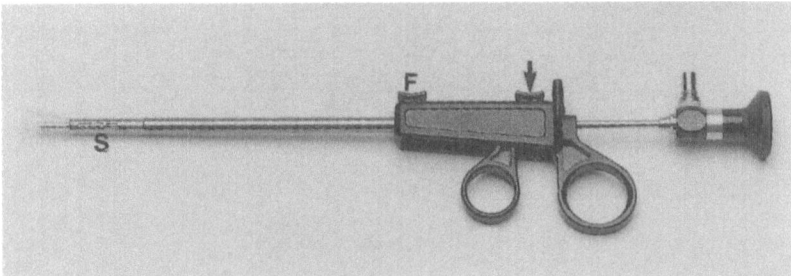

Fig. 5. Endoscopic delivery system. The first safety catch has been depressed, allowing partial stent deployment *(F)*. The second safety catch (→) still needs to be depressed to allow full stent deployment. The side slots can be seen *(S)*. A standard telescope is passed through the introducer to allow visual guidance of stent deployment

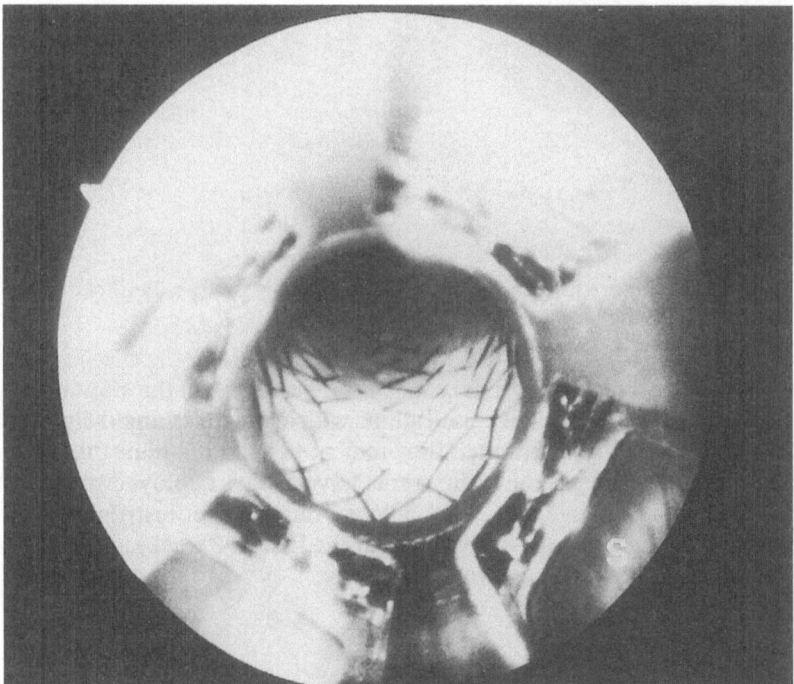

Fig. 6. Endoscopic view through the introducer, the partially deployed stent can be seen, the distal end of the stent being held by the release mechanism until the final safety catch is removed. The position of landmarks such as the verumontanum can be confirmed through the side slots *(S)*

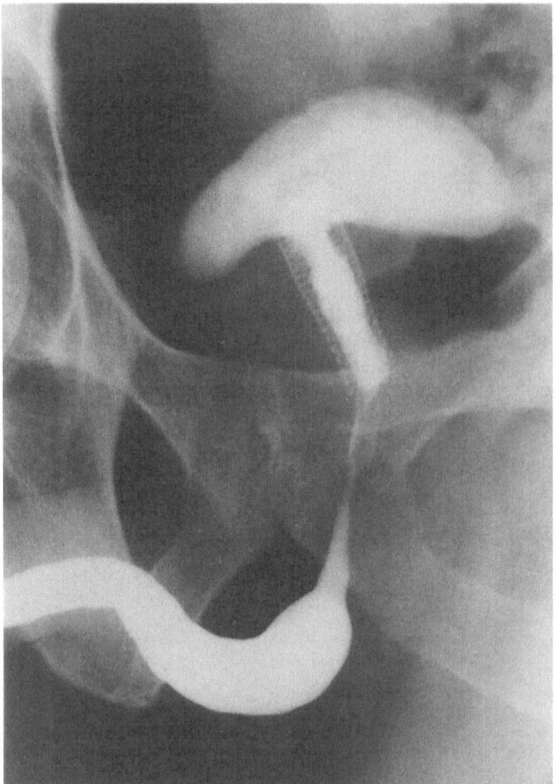

Fig. 7. Ascending urethrogram showing prostatic stent in good position holding open the prostatic urethra

tatic urethra, the second safety lock is depressed, and the stent is fully deployed (Fig. 7). We have used stents with an unconstrained diameter of 14 mm (42 F), and although they may not expand to their full extent within the prostatic lumen, the stents have always deployed to at least 30 F in our experience. This allows endoscopic instrumentation through it, but this must be avoided for the first 2−3 weeks until epithelial covering of the stent is well underway.

Results

We have treated over 95 patients with prostate obstruction. The first patients fell into the high-risk categories for surgery, but we have recently been investigating its use in fitter patients who have requested

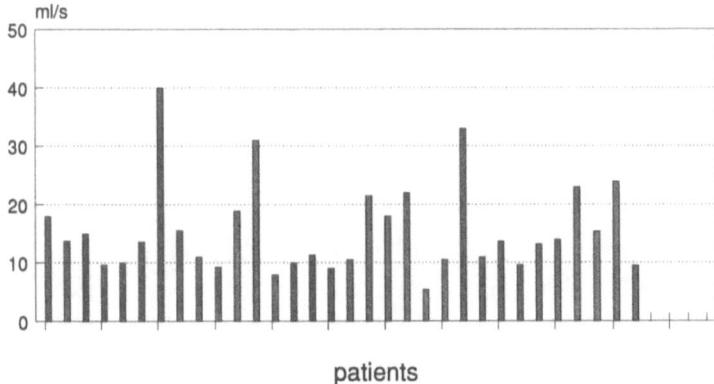

Fig. 8. Histogram demonstrating the improvement in flow rate following stent insertion in patients who presented with urinary retention, ■ post stent insertion

this treatment as an alternative to prostatectomy. Our first 54 patients (mean age 75.7 years; range 49−95) included 34 cases with acute retention, 12 with chronic retention, 4 with severe symptoms and 4 with prostate/Parkinson's disease (48 benign, 6 malignant). In terms of ASA fitness status the distribution was as follows: healthy (1), 3; mild systemic disease (2), 7; severe disease (3), 19; threat to life (4), 25; moribund (5), 0. The technique used was radiological/catheter-mounted device in 24 and endoscopic insertion in 30. The majority of these patients presented in urinary retention with a mean follow-up of 12 (1−28) months showed that 44 patients were passing urine and were fully satisfied with their treatment (Fig. 8−10). The mean post-operative flow rate was 16.6 (5.4−40) ml/s. In those patients with adequate follow-up, the portion of the stent positioned within the prostatic urethra became fully covered with urothelium within 6−9 months. Fifteen patients died of other disease at a mean follow-up of 5.7 (1−23) months.

As with all types of urethral stents, patients experienced some frequency and urgency for 1−3 months, but this persisted only in those patients with intractable detrusor instability. Very few other side effects or complications have been encountered. At endoscopic review we have found that in 12 patients out of 30 followed for more than 9 months there was encrustation on wires which had been left protruding through the bladder neck into the bladder. In an additional two patients with very large diameter prostatic urethras and where the stent had failed to fully expand the lumen, areas of calcification had developed where the wires cross between the lateral lobes. In 3 of these

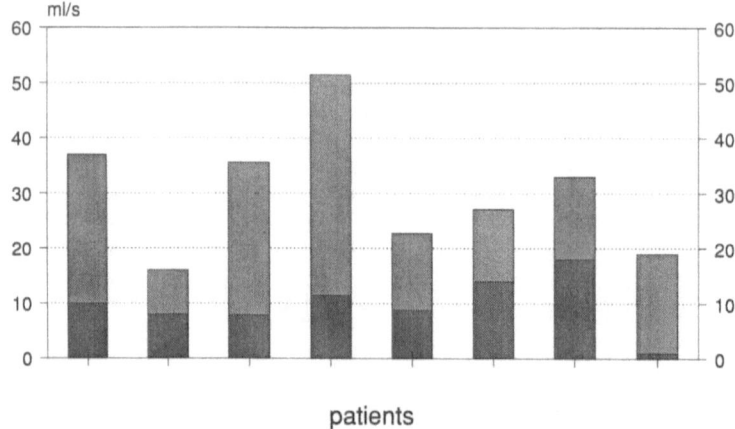

Fig. 9. Histogram demonstrating the improvement in flow rate following stent insertion, in those patients treated for outflow obstruction who were not in urinary retention; ■ before stent insertion, ▨ after stent insertion

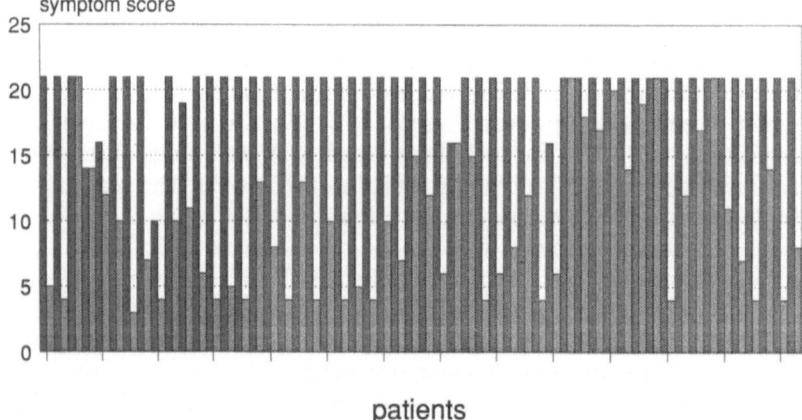

Fig. 10. Histogram demonstrating the improvement in symptom scores following stent insertion; ■ before stent insertion, ▨ after stent insertion

14 patients there was an asymptomatic *Pseudomonas* bacteriuria. The stent can be removed by retrograde displacement back into the bladder followed by either pulling it into a resectoscope sheath or simply pulling it out through the urethra; as the stent is pulled it elongates and narrows, thereby causing little damage to the urethra. We have removed six stents to date, four at up to 1 months and two at 11 months and 18 months after insertion, because of persisting incontinence in patients

with severe recalcitrant detrusor instability, the latter being a patient with Parkinson's disease. In these two patients it was necessary to resect the covering urothelium prior to removal.

Conclusions

There seems to be no doubt that both permanent and temporary prostatic stents have a role in the contemporary management of prostatic obstruction. They are particularly suited to the elderly unfit patient where a major surgical procedure is contraindicated, providing a rapid treatment which can be carried out under local anaesthesia. Although considerably more expensive than temporary stents, permanent stents could potentially provide an alternative to surgical prostatectomy, provided that adequate stent placement can be achieved, thereby avoiding encrustation and the inevitable complications which ensue from this in the long term.

Acknowledgement. I would like to thank E. Milroy for the permission to report the data from the first 54 patients treated at the Middlesex Hospital.

References

1. Moore RA (1935) The morphology of small prostatic carcinoma. J Urol 33:224–234
2. Franks LM (1954) Benign nodular hyperplasia of the prostate: a review. Ann R Coll Surg Engl 14:92–106
3. Glynn RJ, Campion EW, Bouchard GR, Silbert JE (1985) The development of benign prostatic hyperplasia among volunteers in the normative aging study. Am J Epidemiol 121:78–82
4. Mebust WK (1988) Surgical managements of benign prostatic obstruction. Urology [Suppl] 32:12–15
5. Bruskewitz RC, Larsen EH, Madsen PO et al. (1986) Three year follow-up of urinary symptoms after trans-urethral resection of the prostate. J Urol 136:613–615
6. Meyhoff HH (1987) Transurethral versus transvesical prostatectomy: clinical, urodynamic, renographic and enconomic aspects: a randomised study. Scand J Urol Nephrol Suppl 102:1–26
7. Bergman RT, Turner R, Barnes RW et al. (1955) Comparative analysis of one thousand cases of transurethral prostatectomy. J Urol 74:533
8. Chilton CP, Morgan RJ, England HR et al. (1978) A critical evaluation of the results of transurethral resection of the prostate. Br J Urol 50:542–546
9. Roos NP, Ramsey EW (1987) A population based study of prostatectomy: outcomes associated with different surgical procedures. J Urol 137:1184–1188
10. Roos NP, Wennberg JE, Malenka DJ et al. (1989) Mortality and re-operation after open and transurethral resection of the prostate for benign prostatic hyperplasia. N Engl J Med 320:1120–1123

11. Evans JWH, Singer M, Chapple CR, Macartney N, Coppinger SWV, Milroy EJG (1991) Haemodynamic evidence of per-operative cardiac stress during transurethral prostatectomy: preliminary communication. Br J Urol 67:376—380
12. Evans JWH, Singer M, Chapple CR, Macartney N, Coppinger SWV, Milroy EJG (1992) Haemodynamic responses and core temperature changes during transurethral prostatectomy and non-endoscopic general surgical procedures in age matched men. Br Med J 304:666—671
13. Fabian KM (1980) Der interprostatische „partielle Katheter" (urologische Spirale). Urologe 19:236—238
14. Vincente J, Salvador J, Chechile G (1989) Spiral urethral prosthesis as an alternative to surgery in high risk patients with BPH. J Urol 142:1504—1506
15. Fabricius GB, Matz M, Zepnick H (1983) Die Endourethralspirale — eine Alternative zum Dauerkatheter? Z Arztl Fortbild (Jena) 77:482—483
16. Nordling J, Holm HH, Klarskov P, Nielson KK, Andersen JT (1989) Intraprostatic spiral: new device for insertion with patient under local anaesthetic and with ultrasound guidance with three month follow-up. J Urol 142:756—758
17. Harrison NW, De Souza JV (1990) Prostate stenting for outflow obstruction. Br J Urol 65:192—196
18. Nielson KK, Kromann-Andersen B, Nordling J (1989) Relationship between detrusor pressure and urinary flow rate in males with an intra-urethral prostatic spiral. Br J Urol 64:275—279
19. Yachia D (1990) Spontaneous breakage of self-retaining intraprostatic stent. J Urol 144:997—998
20. Nissenkorn I (1989) Experience with a new self retaining intraurethral catheter in patients with urinary retention. J Urol 142:92—94
21. Nissenkorn I, Richter S (1990) A self retaining intra-urethral device. Br J Urol 65:197—200
22. Dobben RL, Wright KC, Dolenz K, Wallace S, Gianturco C (1991) Prostatic urethra dilatation with the Gianturco self-expanding metallic stent: a feasibility study in cadaver specimens and dogs. Am J Roentgenol 156:757—761
23. Parra RO (1991) Titanium urethral stent: an alternative to prostatectomy in the high risk surgical patient. J Urol 145:239A
24. Abrams P, Gillat D, Chadwick D (1991) Intraprostatic stent — experience with the ASI stent to treat bladder outflow obstruction. J Urol 145:373A
25. Holmes SA, Miller PD, Crocker P, Kirby RS (1992) Encrustation of intraprostatic stents — a comparative study. Br J Urol 69:383—387
26. Sigwart U, Puel J, Mirkovitch V et al. (1987) Intravascular stents to prevent occlusion and rectenosis after transluminal angioplasty. N Eng J Med 316:701—706
27. Rousseau H, Puel J, Joffre F et al. (1987) Self-expanding endovascular prosthesis: an experimental study. Radiology 164:709—714
28. Milroy EJG, Chapple CR, Cooper JE, Eldin A, Wallsten H, Seddon AM, Rowles PM (1988) A new treatment for urethral strictures. Lancet 1:1424—1427
29. Sarramon JP, Joffre F, Rischmann P et al. (1989) Prosthese endourethrale Wallstent dans les stenoses recidivantes de l'urethre. Ann Urol 23:383—387
30. Williams G, Jager R, McLoughlin J, El Din A, Machan L, Gill K, Asopa R, Adam A (1989) Use of stents for treating obstruction of urinary outflow in patients unfit for surgery. Br Med J 298:1429
31. Chapple CR, Milroy EJG, Rickards D (1990) Permanently implanted urethral stent for prostatic obstruction in the unfit patient — preliminary report. Br J Urol 66:58—65

Balloon Dilatation of the Prostate

J. A. Vale and R. S. Kirby[1]

Introduction

Benign prostatic hyperplasia (BPH) is a major cause of morbidity amongst elderly men and is reported to have an incidence of 88% amongst men in their 90s [3]. With advances in other fields of medicine and increasing longevity, the number of patients requiring treatment for this complaint will inevitably increase. Already it is estimated that a 50-year-old man has a 20% −25% chance of requiring a prostatectomy during his lifetime [4], and more than 300000 prostatectomies are performed in the United States annually. This represents an enormous financial burden to health services and private insurance companies.

Transurethral prostatectomy (TURP) is the gold standard against which all other treatments must be assessed. There has been recent debate about its relative safety [36], and this has fueled the effort to pursue alternative treatment modalities, including α-adrenoceptor blocking agents [12, 24], 5-α-reductase inhibitors [37], intraprostatic stents [8, 17], microwave hyperthermia [30, 39], and methods of prostatic dilatation. Currently the consensus of opinion is that TURP is safe, with a post-operative mortality rate of only about 0.2%, but does carry an appreciable immediate morbidity rate of 18% [33]. In addition, TURP results in some later complications including post-operative stricture formation in about 3% of patients [34], retrograde ejaculation in a majority of patients [29], and impotence variably reported in the range 4% −40% [5, 16, 20]. Therefore there remains a need to develop and evaluate alternatives to prostatectomy, and the aim of this chapter is to review the current status of balloon dilatation of the prostate.

---

[1] St. Bartholomew's Hospital, Department of Urology, West Smithfield, London EC1A 7BE, UK

History of Prostatic Dilatation

Techniques for the transurethral dilatation of the prostate (TUDP) have been in existence for centuries. However the first instrument developed specifically for this purpose was that described by Guthrie in 1830 (cited in [18]), and shortly after others followed. The next landmark in prostatic dilatation was the procedure of transvesical disruption of the anterior and posterior commisures described by Hollingsworth in 1910 [19]. In this simple technique a small suprapubic cystotomy was made, and the prostate was manually dilated using the index finger. The technique was safer than open prostatectomy and reportedly good results were achieved [13].

In 1956 Deisting [10] introduced a special metal dilator for the prostate that had the advantage over previous systems that it opened within the prostate (Fig. 1) and therefore was not limited in size by urethral access. He reported excellent results in a series of 324 patients; 95% of patients were cured initially and 83%, 74% and 48% were asymptomatic at 3, 5 and 8 years, respectively. However, this study did not compare transurethral dilatation with prostatectomy on a prospective randomized basis, and when such a study was performed within the same centre [1], open prostatectomy and TURP yielded significantly better long-term results and were associated with fewer complications.

TUDP using the technology developed for angioplasty was first reported in 1984 when Burhenne et al. [6] demonstrated that the

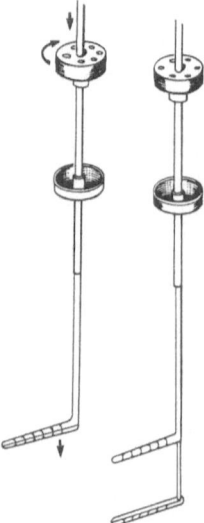

Fig. 1. The Deisting dilator. The dilator blades are separated by turning the upper hand wheel

diameter of the cadaveric male prostatic urethra could be increased by inflating a 24-F balloon within the prostate for 30s. To illustrate the potential value of this finding, Burhenne performed balloon dilatation on his own prostate and recorded an increase in his urinary stream which persisted at 4 weeks. Subsequent studies in dogs [7] demonstrated that a balloon diameter of at least 20mm and an inflation period of 10min were required to produce an increase in urethral diameter which was still present at 14 months. Since then a number of studies of balloon dilatation in patients with BPH have been published.

The Mechanism of Balloon Dilatation of the Prostate

Any successful treatment for BPH must act by reducing the bladder outflow resistance caused by the prostate. There are three main theories as to how TUDP might achieve this. The first is the ischaemic atrophy theory, which proposes that the inflated balloon causes a reduction in blood flow of sufficient duration and magnitude to cause tissue necrosis and subsequent prostatic shrinkage. This mechanism is supported by findings at magnetic resonance imaging (MRI) of an increase in periurethral T2 signal intensity after TUDP, followed by an early return to normal signal intensity and a reduction in prostatic volume in some cases [23]. The prostatic capsule and surrounding tissues appeared normal on all images. However, these MRI findings have not been corroborated by other studies, and histological sections performed on dog prostate immediately after TUDP showed minimal changes apart from some inevitable urothelial denudation [7].

The second proposed mechanism of action of TUDP is that it stretches the prostatic capsule, and that there is some loss of elastic recoil during the procedure. There can be little doubt that capsular stretching does occur on inflation of the balloon; this probably accounts for the pain felt by patients when the procedure is performed under local anaesthesia, and an increase in capsular circumference has been confirmed by performing TUDP on fresh surgical specimens [38]. A loss of elastic recoil is more difficult to prove but would be consistent with the finding that there is often a gradual loss of balloon pressure during dilatation [38].

The final theory is that a successful TUDP produces a disruption of the anterior and/or posterior commissures of the prostate. This was the mechanism of action of the Deisting dilator, and using this instrument there was a characteristic give when disruption occurred. That this may occur during TUDP is beyond doubt; it can be observed cystoscopically [21] and has been suggested as a hallmark of satisfactory dilatation [25].

However, other studies have demonstrated no association between commissurotomy and clinical outcome of TUDP [14, 32].

Thus the mechanism of TUDP remains somewhat controversial. However the apparent success of Hollingsworth's suprapubic prostatic dilatation and the Deisting dilator would be more consistent with the theories of capsular stretching and/or commissurotomy than with the concept of ischaemic atrophy.

The Technique of Transurethral Balloon Dilatation of the Prostate

TUDP can be performed under fluoroscopic or cystoscopic control. The fluoroscopic technique has the advantage that the instrumentation is flexible and therefore lends itself to local anaesthesia. The endoscopic approach has the advantage that the length of balloon can be measured precisely; the verumontanum can be visualized so minimizing the risk of sphincter damage; moreover, the technique is easier for the urologist, who is more familiar with the endoscope than the fluoroscope. We use the Advanced Surgical Intervention (ASI) balloon dilatation catheter system currently, the patients receiving either general or spinal anaesthesia. Antibiotic prophylaxis is not administered routinely unless results of a recent urine culture are unavailable.

The patient is placed in the lithotomy position, and routine cystourethroscopy is performed. The ASI calibration catheter is passed through the instrument channel of the cystoscope, and the 10-ml balloon is inflated and gently withdrawn to the bladder neck. The distance between the bladder neck and external urethral sphincter is measured using the 1-cm markings on the calibration catheter; this determines the length of the prostatic urethra and the appropriate dilatation catheter. The 26-F ASI disposable sheath with obturator is then passed and the obturator removed. The balloon catheter is well lubricated and advanced through the sheath until the first mark on its shaft is visible; this places the distal tip of the catheter in the bladder, and the distal balloon is inflated and snugged down against the bladder neck (Fig. 2). A 0° or 30° telescope is passed through the sheath alongside the catheter, and the sheath withdrawn until the second mark on the catheter is seen. This indicates the distal limit of the balloon, and it should be sited just superior to the sphincter if the urethra has been calibrated correctly. This is confirmed using the telescope. The balloon is inflated to its full diameter of 30 mm (90 F) at 4 atm (Fig. 3) using the positive displacement pump provided. There is a tendency for the balloon to ride up into the bladder during inflation, and this can be prevented by gentle trac-

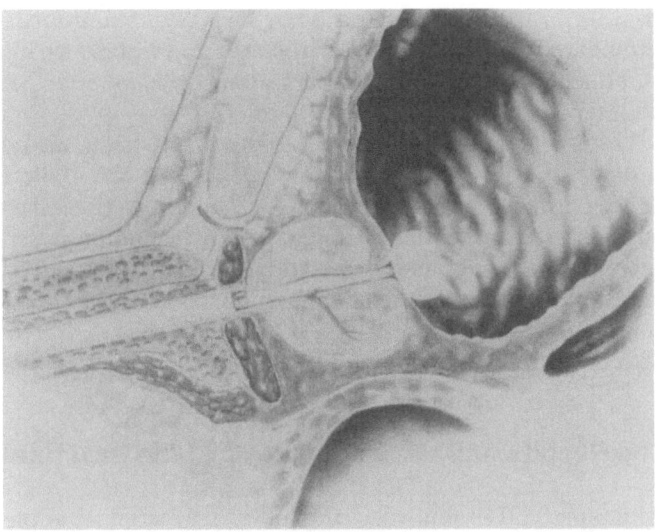

Fig. 2. The dilatation catheter has been positioned accurately

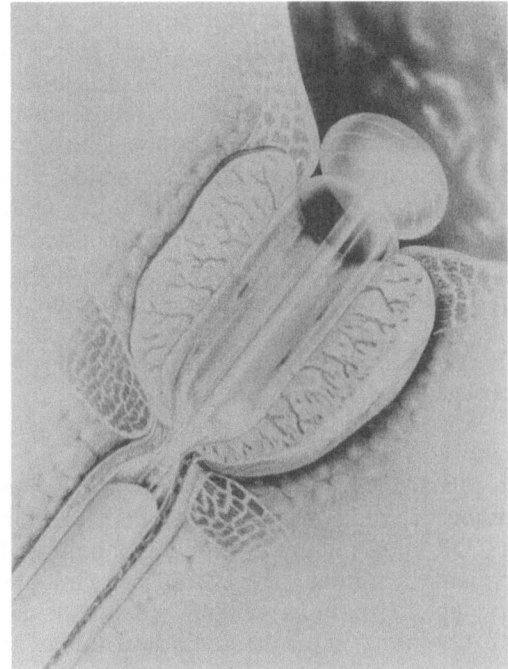

Fig. 3. The balloon has been inflated to a pressure of 3 atm

tion. Its position can be checked by rectal examination. The balloon is left inflated for 10 min and then deflated and withdrawn into the sheath to reduce the chance of urethral trauma on its removal. A 22-F Foley catheter is inserted and left in situ for 72 h.

Using the above technique, there have been no complications amongst the 22 patients we have treated so far. Balloon dilatation under fluoroscopic control can be performed on patients in the supine position. It is essentially similar to the technique described above, except that the sphincter and bladder neck are localized on a urethrogram so permitting urethrographic calibration of the prostatic urethra, and the position of the dilatation balloon is demonstrated by inflation with contrast.

The Results of Balloon Dilatation of the Prostate

Although TUDP is a relatively new technique, multiple case series have been described already with very conflicting results. One of the main factors contributing to this conflict is the difficulty of standardizing the diagnosis of bladder outflow obstruction, and assessing the outcome of intervention objectively. In a large multicentre review of TURP, symptoms were the prime indication for surgery in 91% of cases [33], and in a poll of 89 urologists uroflowmetry was performed in only 8% [22]. Symptoms are not a reliable means of diagnosing obstruction; of 39 patients referred to a urology department with a diagnosis of bladder outflow obstruction, only 61% were obstructed by urodynamic criteria [31]. Furthermore, although a screening peak urinary flow rate of 12 ml/s or less was associated with urodynamic evidence of obstruction in 95% of cases, 35% of patients with symptoms of outflow obstruction and a flow rate of over 12 ml/s were also obstructed by urodynamic criteria. Thus uroflowmetry seems to be fairly specific but not very sensitive in the diagnosis of bladder outflow obstruction.

Some studies of TUDP have assessed efficacy in terms of symptom scores and flow rates, whilst other later studies have included urodynamic data. Perhaps the first comprehensive series was that published by Reddy et al. in 1988 [35], in which 15 patients underwent TUDP using a 25-mm (75-F) balloon under fluoroscopic control. In 8 patients symptoms of "prostatism" were alleviated, with a mean follow-up of 12 months (range 9–16 months). Although it was stated that uroflowmetry improved in these patients, no figures were presented. Results of a larger study from the same centre [38] were published in 1988. On this occasion a total of 70 patients were treated, all of whom had symptoms and signs of moderate or severe prostatism; the series included 7 men in urinary retention. At a mean follow-up of 16.2 months, 46 patients (66%) showed an improvement in their symptom score, an improvement in maximal flow rate, and an insignificant reduction in residual volume. The group of patients who failed to respond included a larger proportion of men with median lobe enlargement, significantly older age, and greater baseline residual volumes. Of the 7 patients in urinary retention, only 2 voided following dilatation.

Many other studies have demonstrated similar results, with a response rate of about 70% in terms of symptomatic improvement, improved flow rates, but poor outcome in cases of acute urinary retention [2, 9, 11, 15]. However, some later studies, particularly those with urodynamic assessment, have been less favourable. Gill et al. [14] reported the results of TUDP using balloons with a diameter of 20 mm or 25 mm in 48 patients with urodynamically confirmed obstruction and 19 patients in urinary retention. Of the former group, less than half reported symptomatic improvement in terms of stream and nocturia, and 89% remained obstructed by urodynamic criteria on repeat cystometrograms 3−11 months after dilatation. The 19 patients in retention fared equally badly; only 3 were able to void, and all were obstructed on cystometric evaluation.

The results of Gill et al. [14] appear dismal compared to some of the studies discussed above, and clearly the reason for this needs consideration. One obvious possibility is that the use of relatively small 20-mm balloons in half of the patients may have skewed the results; there is good evidence that smaller balloons may be ineffective [7, 26]. However a further series has been published recently from the same centre using a massive 35-mm diameter (105F) balloon [32]. Three months following TUDP, 19/27 patients (70%) with bladder outflow obstruction were improved symptomatically and 13/27 patients (48%) were unobstructed by urodynamic criteria. However, this objective benefit from dilatation was short-lived; by 6 months after dilatation only 3 of the 13 patients who had been rendered unobstructed remained so.

The above study by McLoughlin et al. is important. The symptomatic response rate of 70% is similar to that of the most promising studies of TUDP, but not all of the symptomatically improved patients were unobstructed. This illustrates the difficulty of assessing outcome following treatments for benign prostatic hyperplasia and the possible contribution of a placebo response. It is probably unethical to have a sham-operated group in any prospective patient study, although Lepor et al. [28] have compared TUDP to cystoscopy. Klein [25] has compared TUDP with TURP, although the study was not randomized, and a number of exclusion criteria to TUDP were introduced [27]. Thus patients with prostates over 40 g, prominent median lobe hypertrophy, chronic urinary retention or detrusor instability were excluded from the TUDP group. Of those patients fulfilling the selection criteria for TUDP, 64% had a successful outcome on the basis of a greater than 50% reduction in symptoms after the procedure. By the same definition, TURP was successful in 79%. The average weight of resected tissue amongst patients in this successful TURP group was 35 g as compared to 7 g in the patients who had a poor outcome following TURP. It was concluded therefore that TUDP and TURP are really complementary procedures, with TUDP being better for patients with small symptomatic prostates and good bladder function, and TURP remaining the treatment of choice for patients with larger prostates, large residuals or detrusor instability.

Summary

A number of general conclusions can be drawn from the above studies. Firstly, balloon dilatation is a safe procedure, with no serious complications reported in any of the above series. Secondly, it can be expected to alleviate at least some symptoms of "prostatism" in up to 70% of men for 1 year or more and is likely to be especially beneficial in men with small prostates without a prominent median lobe. Most objective evidence to date suggests that TUDP is not a very effective means of relieving obstruction, but then the aim is to treat the patient and not his urodynamic trace; the long-term effects of persisting obstruction are largely unknown. One great advantage of TUDP is that the bladder neck remains intact, and retrograde ejaculation is not a problem. It is of potential value therefore in the treatment of the younger patient with early benign prostatic hyperplasia and a small obstructive prostate.

A final note of caution is necessary. As with many new treatments for BPH, no tissue is taken during TUDP. It is therefore essential to exclude carcinoma of the prostate prior to treatment by digital rectal examination, prostate specific antigen and/or transrectal ultrasound with ultrasound-guided biopsy. The patient must be informed also that he may require a prostatectomy in the future if balloon dilatation is unsuccessful in the longer term.

References

1. Aalkjaer V (1965) Transurethral resection/prostatectomy versus dilatation treatment in hypertrophy of the prostate: II. A comparison of the late results. Urol Int 20:17−22
2. Baert L, Werbrouck P, Bamelis B et al. (1991) Balloon dilatation of the prostate. Urol Int 47:74−76
3. Berry SJ, Coffey DS, Walsh PC et al. (1984) The development of human benign prostatic hyperplasia with age. J Urol 132:474−479
4. Birkhoff JJ (1983) Natural history of benign prostatic hypertrophy. In: Hinman F (ed) Benign prostatic hypertrophy. Springer, Berlin Heidelberg New York
5. Bruskewitz RC, Larsen EH, Madsen P et al. (1986) 3-Year follow-up of urinary symptoms after transurethral resection of the prostate. J Urol 136:613−615
6. Burhenne HJ, Chisholm RJ, Quenville NF (1984) Prostatic hyperplasia: radiological intervention. Radiology 152:655−657
7. Castaneda F, Lund G, Larson BW et al. (1987) Prostatic urethra: experimental dilation in dogs. Radiology 163:645−648
8. Chapple CR, Milroy EJG, Rickards D (1990) Permanently implanted urethral stent for prostatic obstruction in the unfit patient. Br J Urol 66:58
9. Daughtry JD, Rodan BA, Bean WJ (1990) Balloon dilatation of prostatic urethra. Urology 36:203−209
10. Deisting W (1956) Transurethral dilatation of the prostate: a new method in the treatment of prostatic hypertrophy. Urol Int 2:158−171
11. Dowd JB, Smith JJ (1990) Balloon dilatation of the prostate. Urol Clin North Am 17:671−677
12. Fabricius PG, Weizert P, Dunzendorfer U et al. (1990) A randomized double-blind placebo controlled trial on the efficacy of once a day terazasin in benign prostatic hyperplasia. Prostate 3:85
13. Franck O (1938) Die Sprengung des Prostataringes. Münch Med Wochenschr 85:777−782
14. Gill KP, Machan LS, Allison DJ, Williams G (1989) Bladder outflow tract obstruction from benign prostatic hypertrophy treated by balloon dilatation. Br J Urol 64:618−622
15. Goldenberg SL, Perez-Marrero RA, Lee LM, Emerson L (1990) Endoscopic balloon dilatation of the prostate: early experience. J Urol 144:83−87
16. Hargreave TB, Stephenson TP (1977) Potency and prostatectomy. Br J Urol 49:683
17. Harrison NW, DeSouza JV (1990) Prostatic stenting for outflow obstruction. Br J Urol 65:192
18. Hinman F (ed) (1983) Benign prostatic hypertrophy. Springer, Berlin Heidelberg New York, Chap 5
19. Hollingsworth E (1910) Dilatation of the prostatic urethra for the relief of the symptoms of prostatic enlargement. Ann Surg 51:597−599
20. Holtgrewe HL, Valk WL (1964) Late results of transurethral prostatectomy. J Urol 92:51
21. Isorna S, Maynar M, Belon JL et al. (1989) Prostatic urethroplasty: endoscopic findings. Semin Intervent Radiol 6:46−56
22. Iverson P, Bruskewitz K, Jensen ME, Madsen PO (1983) Transurethral prostatic resection in the treatment of prostatism with high urinary flow. J Urol 129:995−997
23. Johnson SD, Kuni CC, Castaneda F et al. (1987) MR imaging of patients undergoing prostatic balloon dilatation. Radiology 165:332

24. Kirby RS, Coppinger SWC, Corcoran M et al. (1987) Prazosin in the treatment of prostatic obstruction. Br J Urol 60:136
25. Klein LA (1991) Balloon dilatation of the prostate as compared with transurethral resection of the prostate for treatment of benign prostatic hypertrophy. World J Urol 9:29–31
26. Klein LA, Lemming B (1989) Balloon dilatation for prostatic obstruction. Urology 33:198–201
27. Klein LA, Perez-Marrero RA, Bowers GW et al. (1990) Transurethral cystoscopic balloon dilatation of the prostate. J Endourol 4:183–191
28. Lepor H, Sypherd D, Machi G, Denis J (1991) Randomized double-blind study comparing the effectiveness of balloon dilatation of the prostate and cystoscopy for the treatment of symptomatic benign prostatic hyperplasia. J Urol 145:362A
29. Libman E, Fichten CB (1987) Prostatectomy and sexual function. Urology 29:467
30. Lindner A, Golomb J, Lev A (1987) Local hyperthermia of the prostate gland for the treatment of BPH and urinary retention. Br J Urol 60:567
31. McLoughlin J, Gill KP, Abel PD, Williams G (1990) Symptoms versus flow rates versus urodynamics in the selection of patients for prostatectomy. Br J Urol 66:303–305
32. McLoughlin J, Keane PF, Jager R et al. (1991) Dilatation of the prostatic urethra with a 35 mm balloon. Br J Urol 67:177–181
33. Mebust WK, Holtgrewe HL, Cockett ATK et al. (1989) Transurethral prostatectomy: immediate and postoperative complications. A cooperative study of 13 participating institutions evaluating 3885 patients. J Urol 141:243–247
34. Mebust WK, Holtgrewe HL (1989) Current status of transurethral prostatectomy: a review of the AUA National Cooperative Study. World J Urol 6:194–197
35. Reddy PK, Wasserman N, Castaneda F, Castaneda-Zuniga WR (1988) Balloon dilatation of the prostate for treatment of benign prostatic hyperplasia. Urol Clin North Am 15:529–535
36. Roos NP, Wennberg JE, Malenka DJ et al. (1989) Mortality and reoperation after open and transurethral resection of the prostate for benign prostatic hyperplasia. N Engl J Med 320:1120–1124
37. Stoner E (1990) The clinical development of a 5-α-reductase inhibitor, finasteride. J Steroid Biochem 37:375
38. Wasserman NF, Reddy PK, Zhang G et al. (1990) Experimental treatment of benign prostatic hyperplasia with transurethral balloon dilatation of the prostate: preliminary study in 73 humans. Radiology 177:485–494
39. Yerushalmi A, Fishelovitz Y, Singer D et al. (1985) Localized deep microwave hyperthermia in the treatment of poor operative risk patients with benign prostatic hyperplasia. J Urol 133:873

Urodynamic Studies Before and After Transurethral Balloon Dilatation of the Prostate

P. De Geeter, W. Holtermann, and H.-J. Melchior[1]

The technique of transurethral balloon dilatation of the prostate (TUDP) in patients with benign prostatic hypertrophy is very appealing considering the simplicity of the method and the possibility of performing the procedure under local anesthesia. Even if the long-term effectiveness of the method is still uncertain as compared to a standard transurethral resection of the prostate (TURP), many studies report significant relief of symptoms in approximately 60% of the patients with pure lateral lobe hyperplasia [2]. In these cases relief of obstruction has been reported up to now only in terms of symptom score improvement and/or peak flow changes. In our protocol data from pressure-flow measurements have been used for the selection and evaluation of patients.

Technique

We have been performing TUDP in our department since September 1989. In our approach we slightly modified the technique described by Castaneda et al. [1] and performed the procedure under local anesthesia as described earlier. At the beginning of the procedure, cystoscopy is performed to determine the length of the prostatic urethra and to assess the size of the median lobe, if one exists. Prior to the removal of the cystoscope a guide wire is passed into the bladder. The further procedure is then monitored under fluoroscopic control. The external sphincter can be located exactly at this moment by retrograde urethrography. The dilating balloon (Boston Scientific) has a usable length of 4 cm and has radiopaque markers at each end. The pressure balloon is placed in the prostatic urethra in such a way that the proximal marker

---

[1] Städtische Kliniken Kassel, Urologische Abteilung, Mönckebergstraße 41, W-3500 Kassel, FRG

on the catheter is lying just distal to the external sphincter. The balloon is inflated to its full diameter of 30 mm (90-F) exerting 3 atm (45 PSI) pressure on the prostate. In most cases powerful traction must be applied during initial inflation to overcome the tendency of the catheter to slip forward into the bladder. The balloon is deflated and removed after 10 min. A repeat urethrogram is then performed to assess the state of the urethra and the bladder neck region. Bleeding is fairly common, and in all cases a 22-F Foley catheter is inserted for continuous bladder irrigation. Generally this catheter remains in place for 12–24 h.

Material and Methods

All patients in our study were primarily selected for transurethral resection of the prostate according to the department's routine, which always includes history, physical examination, digital rectal examination, serum prostatic specific antigen, sonography, and cystoscopy. A total of 32 patients, with a mean age of 73 years ($\pm$ 8.5), entered our study and underwent transurethral balloon dilatation of the prostate as an alternative to standard TURP. Of our patients 15% entered the hospital with an acute urinary retention and exactly 50% of the patients had residuals of more than 100 ml (Table 1).

For the purpose of this study, history included a symptom score analysis according to the Madsen point system [3]. In addition, all

Table 1. Indications ($n = 32$)

Indication	n	%
Acute urinary retention[a]	5	15.6
Residual urine >250 ml	6	18.75
Residual urine 100–250 ml	10	31.25
Residual rine <100 ml	11	34.4

[a] Includes two patients with detrusor acontractility

Table 2. Preoperative parameters ($n = 32$)

Parameter	Mean/median (range)
Score (Madsen)	16.3/16.0 (10–23) points
Peak flow (Q_{max})	5.3/5.2 (0–14) ml/s
Residual urine	199/145 (0–600) ml
Detrusor pressure	102/100 (0–165) cm H_2O

patients underwent further urodynamic evaluation preoperatively, including repeated uroflowmetry, if possible, and a pressure-flow study.

All patients had a symptom score of at least 10; the average was 16, and the peak urinary flow rate averaged 5.3 ml/s. Two patients with acute retention were found to have detrusor acontractility during the pressure-flow study. All other patients had elevated detrusor pressures at maximum flow with a mean pressure of 100 cm H_2O (Table 2).

Symptom scores, flow rates, and postvoiding residuals were reassessed within 2 weeks after TUDP and during later follow-up after 3, 6, and 12 months, respectively. Additional pressure-flow studies were performed at later follow-up in 27 of the 32 patients.

Results

For the assessment of the postoperative results the patients were grouped according to percentage improvement in peak uroflow and symptom score and according to their postvoiding residuals. TUDP was considered successful if the symptom score and the flow rate improved more than 50%, provided the postvoiding residual was less than 50 ml. The outcome was considered satisfactory if a 50% improvement of only one parameter was observed. The outcome of all other patients were classified as no-change or poor. According to this classification the treatment was successful initially in 25% of the patients (8/32) and satisfactory in another 28% (9/32). The procedure was not successful in 47% of the cases (11/32).

A detailed analysis of the symptom scores reveals a 78% improvement of the mean symptom score after successful treatment and a 66% improvement in those patients with a satisfactory result. The mean score decreased from 16.1 in both groups to 3.5 and 5.4, respectively. A total lack of symptomatic improvement was found in the third group (Table 3).

Postoperative flow rates increased significantly after a successful treatment. The mean preoperative flow rate was 4.8 ml/s in this group

Table 3. Symptoms scores ($n = 32$): mean/median (range)

Outcome	Preoperative	Postoperative
Successful ($n = 8$)	16.1/16 (10−22)	3.5/4.0 (0−8)
Satisfactory ($n = 9$)	16.1/16 (10−20)	5.4/5.0 (2−11)
No change/poor ($n = 15$)	16.6/16 (12−23)	15.4/16 (6−23)

Table 4. Uroflowmetry ($n = 32$): mean/median (range)

Outcome	Preoperative	Postoperative
Successful ($n = 8$)	4.8/5.2 (0–8.1)	13.5/12.7 (7.5–25)
Satisfactory ($n = 9$)	8.6/9.0 (1–14)	11.7/12.0 (6–18)
No change/poor ($n = 15$)	3.6/4.0 (0–9.3)	3.8/2.0 (0–14)

and improved promptly with balloon dilatation to 13.5 ml/s postoperatively (181% !). In the group of patients who experienced satisfactory treatment the postoperative increase in flow rates was not significant, with a mean increase of only 36%, or 3.1 ml/s (Table 4).

The symptom scores at later follow-up showed that most patients remained symptom free up to 1 year after a successful or satisfactory treatment (Fig. 1). Only two patients − one in each group − did not sustain their initial improvement, and symptoms returned after 3 and 6 months, respectively.

Some objective evidence for the symptomatic improvement in these groups is given by the flow rate pattern at later follow-up. In some cases improvement is clearly visible and long lasting. Although most patients had preoperative flow rates greater than 5 ml/s, it is interesting to note that two patients with acute urinary retention were treated successfully. In many other patients, however, the increase in flow rate was not so dramatic at closer observation (Fig. 2).

After successful or satisfactory dilatation postvoiding residuals decreased significantly compared to preoperative values. On the other hand, postoperative pressure-flow studies, which were performed in 27 of 32 patients revealed no significant change in mean detrusor pressure at later follow-up. As a matter of fact, most patients who experienced a „successfull" dilatation were found to have constant elevated voiding pressures postoperatively, with a mean detrusor pressure of 106 cm H_2O (Table 5).

In the group of patients who were dilated successfully, a prompt decrease in the detrusor pressure was observed only once postoperatively. For all other patients in this group there was even a tendency towards more elevated pressures at later follow-up (Fig. 3a). Occasionally a clearly visible and sustained decrease in detrusor pressure was seen, elthough this occurred almost exclusively in the group of patients in whom the outcome of the dilatation procedure was only „satisfactory" and not the very best (Fig. 3b). In these cases the presumed relief of obstruction did not correspond with the clinical result of the treatment. After 1 year of follow-up 9 patients (28%) had sustained their

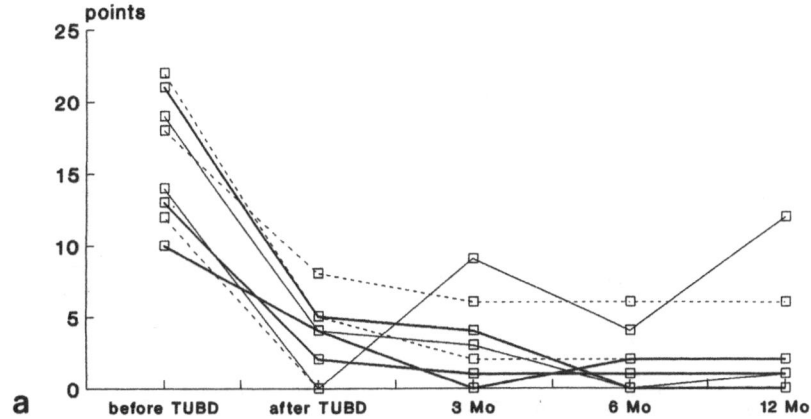

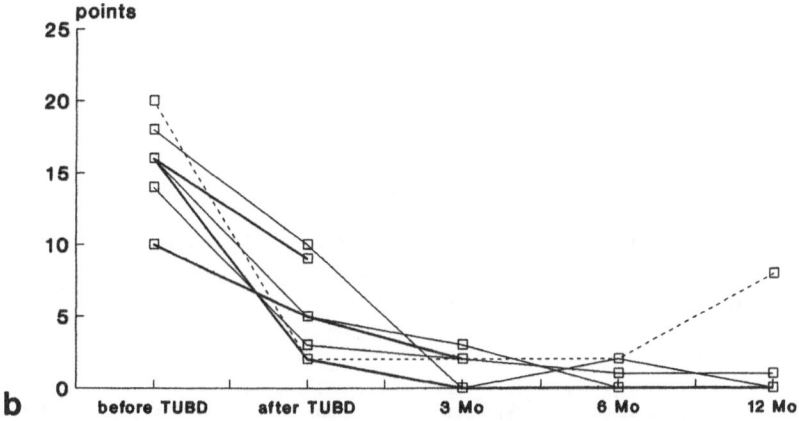

Fig. 1a, b. Symptom scores. **a** Successful cases. **b** Satisfactory cases

initial improvement and were still very satisfied. A total of 14 patients (43.8%) was not satisfied at all, and 11 of these had TURP within 6 weeks after dilatation of the prostate (Table 6).

Discussion

In our experience TUDP had a rather low success rate compared to standard TURP. Only one-third of our patients experienced a significant improvement without clear evidence that the outlet obstruction had been relieved.

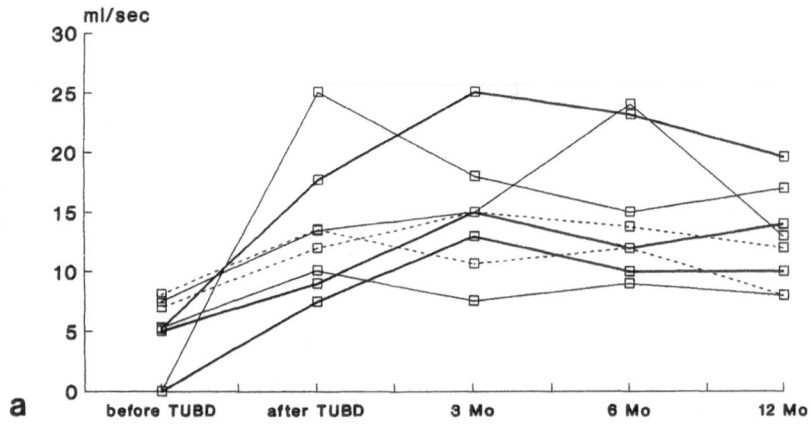

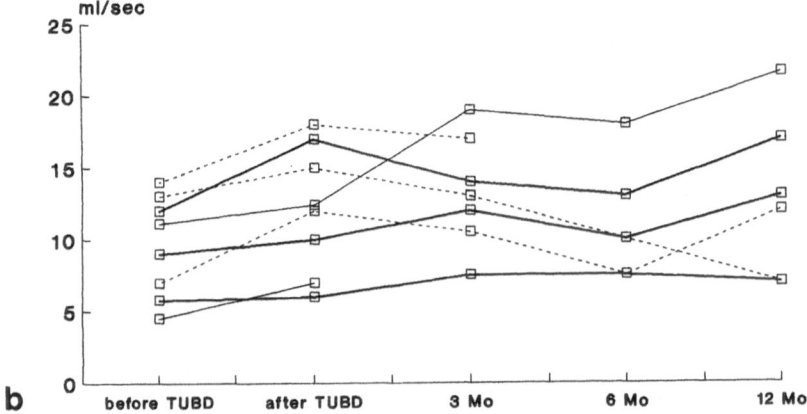

Fig. 2a, b. Uroflowmetry. **a** Successful cases. **b** Satisfactory cases

Table 5. Detrusor pressure ($n = 27$): mean/median (range)

Outcome	Preoperative	Postoperative
Successful ($n = 7$)	122/125 (75−164)	106/105 (65−152)
Satisfactory ($n = 9$)	102/100 (60−140)	107/110 (75−140)
No change/poor ($n = 11$)	90/ 90 (0−165)	85/ 75 (0−140)

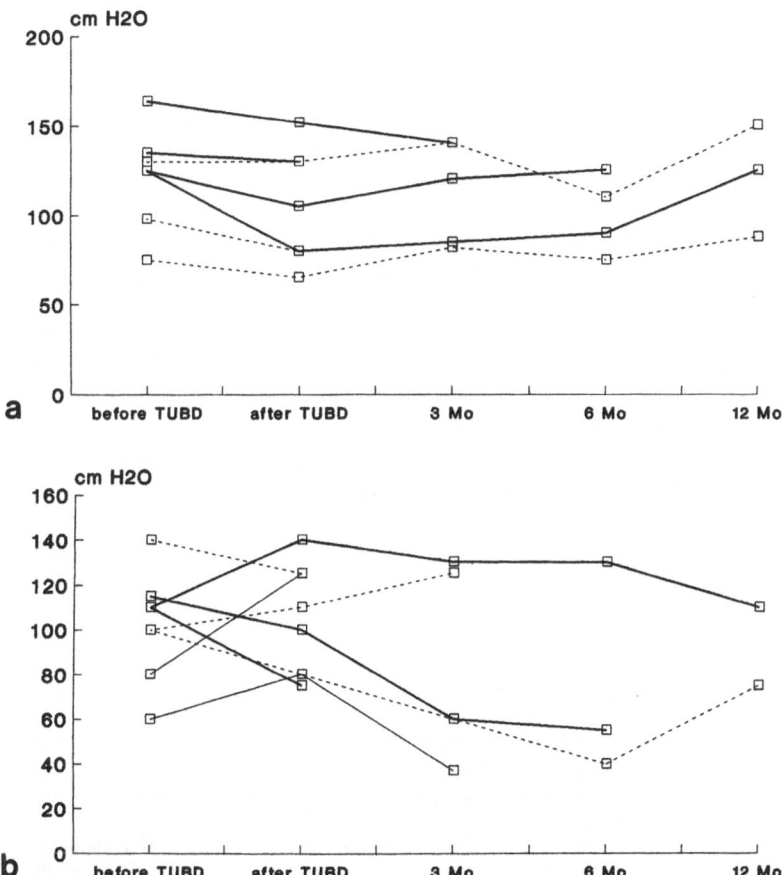

Fig. 3a, b. Detrusor pressure. **a** Successful cases. **b** Satisfactory cases

Table 6. Results at 1-year follow-up ($n = 32$)

	n	%
Subjective outcome		
Very satisfied	9	28
Satisfied	2	6.25
Not satisfied	3	9.4
Subsequent TURP		
Within 6 weeks after TUDP	11	34.4
At 12 months after TUDP	1	3.2
Lost to follow-up within 3 months	6	18.75

We have been performing TUDP under local anesthesia, which is not sufficient in most cases, and additional pain medication is almost always necessary. TUDP is a painful procedure, and if we must perform balloon dilatation in the future, we would recommend spinal or general anesthesia. As an alternative we could of course try the effectiveness of a regional paraprostatic block, as described by Reddy in 1990 [4].

One must also recall that this lind of treatment is rather expensive, and that each dilatation catheter costs (in Germany) approximately U.S.$ 600.

The key of the problem may be that one must select the patients properly. However, in our experience it seems very difficult at the moment to predict the outcome of the procedure. On the other hand, we do not know at present how to interpret the urodynamic results. In this series we could not demonstrate clear-cut evidence for the relief of outlet obstruction after „successful" balloon dilatation.

References

1. Castaneda F, Reddy P, Wasserman N, Hulbert J, Lund G, Letourneau JG, Hunter DW, Castaneda Zuniga WR, Amplatz K (1987) Benign prostatic hypertrophy: retrograde transurethral dilation of the prostatic urethra in humans. Radiology 163:649
2. Hulbert JC, Reddy PK, Castaneda F, Ercole CJ, Zhang G, Hernandez Graulau JM, Castaneda WR, Letourneau JG, Wasserman N, Hunter DW (1989) Transurethral dilatation of the prostate (prostatic „divulsion") − mechanism of action and results. J Urol 141:253A
3. Madsen PO, Iversen P (1983) A point system for selecting operative candidates. In: Hinman F Jr (ed) Benign prostatic hyperplasia. Springer, Berlin Heidelberg New York, pp 763−765
4. Reddy PK (1990) A new technique to anesthetize the prostate for transurethral balloon dilatation of the prostate gland. Urol Clin North Am 17:55−56

Hyperthermia or Thermotherapy of Benign Prostatic Hyperplasia: What Is the Difference?

R. Harzmann and D. Weckermann[1]

There is a very strong tendency — especially in connection with benign prostatic hyperplasia (BPH) — to substitute operative procedures with nonoperative or minimally invasive techniques. Examples are balloon dilatation, intraprostatic devices, wall stents, transurethral incision (TUIP), and the use of transurethral lasers (TULIP). Lately, these therapeutic measures have fallen a little behind and are being partially overtaken by thermal treatment modalities of BPH. For the past 2 years this technique first described in 1985 by Yerushalmi et al. [27], has fascinated patients, media, and parts of the medical community. This led to publications praising local hyperthermia of BPH as an effective and side-effect-free alternative therapy and thus superior to the well-known operative techniques [3, 4, 18−20, 23, 25, 27].

Hyperthermia/Thermotherapy Machines

Currently, ten machines for transrectal or transurethral hyperthermia/thermotherapy are available. Newer machines have the dual capability for either transrectal or transurethral application of heat. Table 1 shows names, manufacturers, routes of application, and special technical details. In general, microwaves are used for the treatment. Only one machine (Thermex II) works with mixed frequencies [20, 24], the lowest of which (0.5 MHz) is within the longwave range. The goal is a tissue temperature of 43 °C, which is controlled by transrectal or transurethral thermocouples, or which are only calculated. All machines contain elaborate computer systems to ensure induction, maintenance, and control of the temperature in the target organ. This is part of the reason for the high cost, between 300 000 and 400 000 DM. The only

[1] Urologische Klinik, Zentralklinikum Augsburg, Stenglinstraße, W-8900 Augsburg 1, FRG

Table 1. Technology and application modalities of prostate hyperthermia machines
(Prostatron = thermotherapy apparatus)

Appliance/Company	Route	Frequency	Cooling	Modalities
Prostathermer/Biodan	Rectal	915 MHz	+	$5-10 \times 1$ h
Promeditech/Biodan	Rectal	915 MHz	+	$5-10 \times 1$ h
Primus/Tecnomatix	Rectal	915 MHz	+	$5-10 \times 1$ h
Curamed/Aquadent	Rectal	?	−	$5-10 \times 1$ h
Prostek 3000/Clinitherm	Rectal	915 MHz	−	1×1 h
BSD 50/BSD-Med. Corp.	Urethral	434 MHz	−	$5-10 \times 1$ h
Thermex II/Direx	Urethral	0.5 MHz	−	1×3 h
Prostatron/Technomed	Urethral	1296 MHz	+	1×1 h
Prostcare/Bruker	Urethral/rectal	915 MHz	+	1×1 h
Microfocus 500/Medi-Therm	Urethral/rectal	915 MHz	−/+	$5-10 \times 1$ h

exception is the Curamed; this office unit costs about 6000 DM, the home version about 600 DM. Noteworthy is that these units do not use microwave or longwave current but function as an immersion heater. The cost of the thermotherapy machine Prostatron is 1 000 000 DM. The technique of this unit is not based on local hyperthermia but on much higher temperatures within the prostate gland (45°−60°C).

This kind of treatment is always ambulatory. The time required is about 1−3 h. The duration of the total treatment about 5−6 weeks; depending on the device used, up to ten sessions are necessary.

Results of BPH Hyperthermia

The publications to date view the effects of prostate hyperthermia preponderantly as positive. This corresponds with the manufacturer's statement of a „revolutionary breakthrough" in the therapy of BPH. The fact that placebo effects, especially in the treatment of BPH, play an important role, however, must be kept in mind [2] (placebo success rates >30%). For this reason a critical evaluation of the hyperthermia data is in order [8].

Subjective positive results after hyperthermia are reported in 58%−90% [3, 4, 18−20, 25] and objective results in between 7.1% [26] and 83% [19]. It is notable that different authors have differing definitions of the term „objective". Truly objective parameters are *repeated* controls of uroflow and postvoiding residuals in conjunction with prostate volumetry and histological check-up. With the application of hard parameters (prostate volumetry, histology) it was noted that local prostate hyperthermia has no measurable effect on the prostate (Table 2). Changes in prostate volume or histological changes, as a result of local

Table 2. Prostate volumetry and histology after local BPH hyperthermia

Reference	Year	Volume	Histology
Braf et al. [5]	1990	Unchanged	0
Leib et al. [18]	1991	Unchanged	Inflammation
Meshorer [20]	1990	–	Glandular atrophy[a]
Rigatti et al. [22]	1989	–	Inflammation (PC[b]: necroses)
Sapozink et al. [23]	1990	Unchanged	Inflammation
Strohmaier et al. [26]	1990	Unchanged	Inflammation

[a] Experimental findings.
[b] Prostate cancer.

transrectal or transurethral hyperthermia, are not be found. At best, one finds nonspecific changes, for example, edema or moderate inflammation reactions.

Thus, it is not surprising that a recent publication states that only 2 out of 28 patients treated with transrectal hyperthermia for BPH showed objective improvement in the control parameters. With a success rate of 7.1%, these results clearly show less success than those achieved with placebos only [26].

The discrepancy between good subjective and poor objective treatment results is thus evidently due to placebo effects [8]. Furthermore, it seems possible that local microwave hyperthermia of BPH induces functional disabilities of the bladder neck and intraprostatic alphareceptors [12, 13]. Consequently, the effects of local hyperthermia should be compared only to the effects pf pharmacotherapy with alpha-blockers and not to those of the operative therapy of BPH, which still is the most effective form of BPH treatment [12, 13].

Definition of Local Hyperthermia

Local hyperthermia has been an entity in oncology for years. This therapy operates with tissue temperatures between 42° and 44°C, the optimum being 43°C. It is necessary to point out that the effectiveness of local warming shows a dose-time relationship. Effects on malignant tissue cannot be shown if the temperature does not reach its therapeutic value of 43°C (Fig. 1). A remarkable fact of local hyperthermia is that malignant and normal tissue show different temperature sensibility [10, 11]. Temperatures of 43°C cause at least partial definitive damage to malignant tissue, whereas no lasting damage occurs in normal tissue [10]. Thus, definitive effects of local hyperthermia in benign conditions, such as BPH, the first cannot be expected from [12, 13].

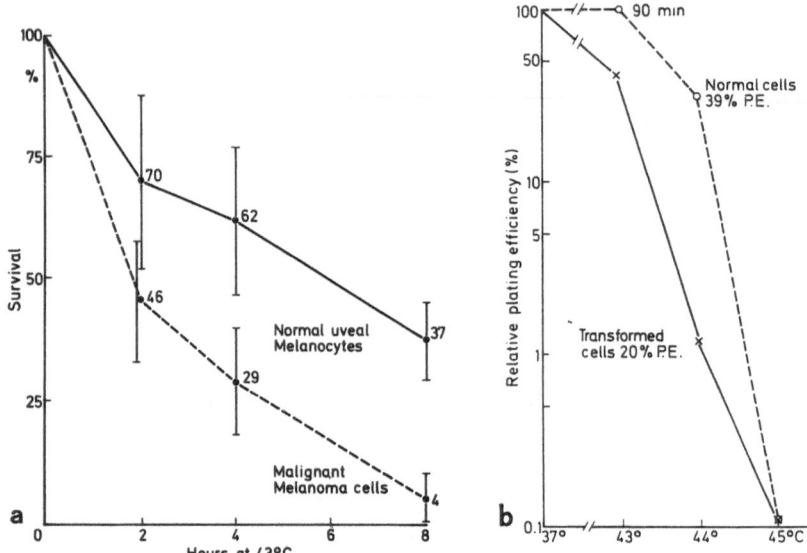

Fig. 1a, b. Different temperature susceptibility of normal and tumorous tissue. **a** Temperature dependence of the damage of normal cells and malignant transformed cells. **b** Definitive damage of normal and malignant cells, starting at 45°C [6]

Although not as a monotherapeutic measure, local hyperthermia could, on the other hand, favorably influence the localized carcinoma of the prostate and of the bladder (Fig. 2) [9, 16, 17]. A basis for this is the homogeneous distribution of heat throughout the entire prostate. Since the currently available hyperthermia machines (exception: Thermex II) use microwaves between 434 and 915 MHz, and, at the same time, these frequencies show a poor penetration of energy, these machines appear unacceptable for this indication. Frequencies from 0.3 to 8.0 MHz are needed since these are capable of homogeneous distribution of energy throughout the tissue [10–15, 21]. In contrast, microwave therapy leads to a radial temperature gradient of 4°–7°C per centimeter of tissue [1], and thus a steep drop in temperature from therapeutic into the ineffective ranges, occurs within the prostate.

Definition of Thermotherapy

The group of Devonec [7] uses tissue temperatures of 45°–60°C. This takes into account the fact that normal and tumor tissue show definitive changes in cell structures beyond 45°C (Fig. 3). The machine developed

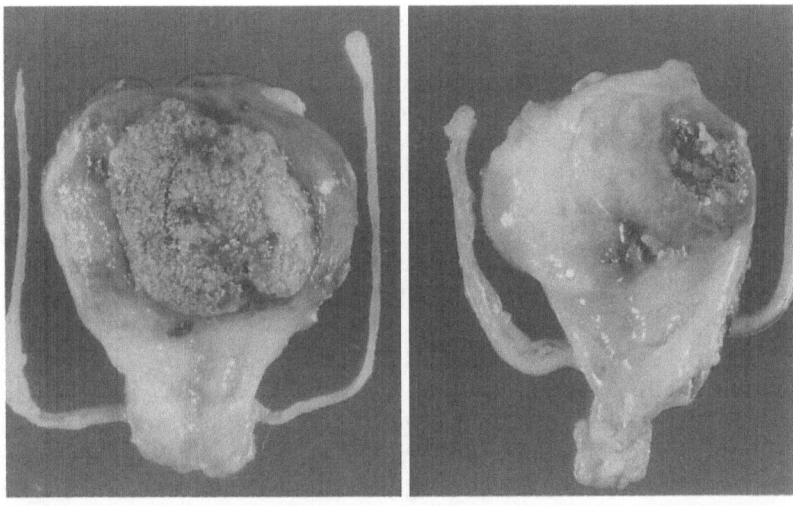

Fig. 2a, b. Local hyperthermia of an experimental urinary bladder tumor (rabbit). **a** Untreated tumor. **b** Tumor treated with local hyperthermia. After local hyperthermia there is a subtotal tumor reduction (tumor volume substantially reduced as compared with the nontreated carcinoma). The normal tissue shows no evidence of hyperthermia-induced changes

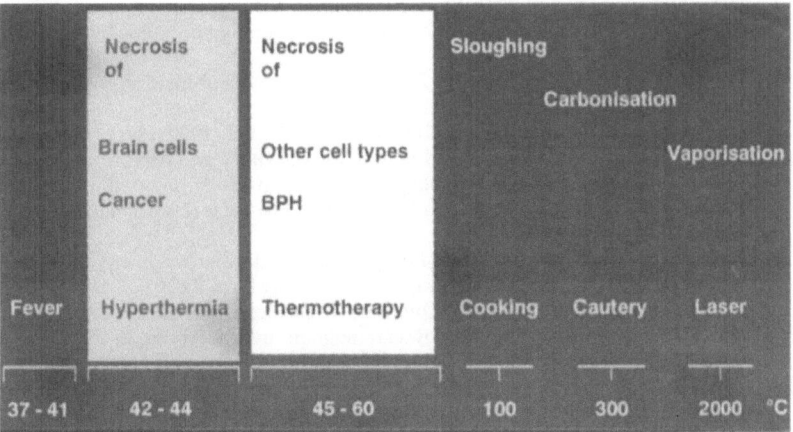

Fig. 3. Definition of various temperature ranges and their effects on different tissues

by this group also uses microwaves (1296 MHz) but has a much higher energy power, thus inducing temperatures of 60°–80°C in the direct vicinity of the transurethral zone of application. To prevent resulting damage to the prostatic urethra, a computer-controlled cooling system was developed for this part of the urethra. A further advantage is that pain in the urethra is avoided, and the treatment can be performed without anesthesia.

As a consequence of such local thermotherapy of BPH a reduction in prostate volume of about 30% of the patients was shown. On the other hand, however, it was found that this procedure leads to necroses of prostate tissue.

The goal of thermotherapy in BPH is to compete with the standard therapy of BPH – transurethral resection – with avoidance of the operative treatment and its consequence – retrograde ejaculation.

Further clinical studies are needed to determine whether thermotherapy is capable of replacing transurethral resection as the gold standard of BPH therapy. Furthermore, it is necessary to check whether this therapeutic modality holds advantages for the patient with a localized cancer of the prostate, who, secondary to a reduced general appearance, cannot be treated curatively (radical prostatectomy).

References

1. Astrahan MA, Sapozink MD, Luxton G, Kampp TD, Petrovich Z (1989) Microwave applicator for transurethral hyperthermia of benign prostatic hyperplasia. Int J Hyperthermia 5:37–51
2. Ball AJ, Feneley RCL, Abrams PH (1981) The natural history of untreated „prostatism". Br J Urol 53:613–616
3. Bichler K-H, Strohmaier WL, Steimann J, Flüchter SH (1990) Hyperthermia in urology. In: Gautherie M (ed) Interstitial, endocavitary and perfusional hyperthermia. Springer, Berlin Heidelberg New York, pp 43–58
4. Bichler K-H (1988) Mikrowellentherapie bei Prostataerkrankungen. Niere-Blase-Prostata 4:18–19
5. Braf ZF, Saranga R, Matzkin H (1990) Local deep microwave hyperthermia treatment for BPH – follow-up in 132 patients. Eur Urol 18:107
6. Chen TT, Heidelberger C (1969) Quantitative studies on the malignant transformation of mouse prostate cells by carcinogenic hydrocarbons in vitro. Int J Cancer 4:166–174
7. Devonec M, Berger N, Bringeon G, Carter S, Perrin P (1991) Long-term histological effects of transurethral microwave therapy (TUMT) on benign prostatic hypertrophy. J Urol 145:363A
8. Fabricius PG, Schäfer J, Schmeller N, Chaussy C (1991) Efficacy of transrectal hyperthermia for benign prostatic hyperplasia: a placebo-controlled study. J Urol 145:363A
9. Gottlieb CF, Seibert GB, Block NL (1988) Interaction of irradiation and microwave-induced hyperthermia in the Dunning R 3327G prostatic adenocarcinoma model. Radiology 169:243–247

10. Harzmann R (1980) Hochfrequenz-Hyperthermie beim Harnblasenkarzinom. Urban and Schwarzenberg, Baltimore
11. Harzmann R, Bichler K-H, Gericke D (1988) Transurethrale lokale Hochfrequenz-Hyperthermie des Harnblasenkarzinoms. In: Bichler KH, Flüchter SH, Strohmaier WL (eds) Therapie des Harnblasenkarzinoms. Springer, Berlin Heidelberg New York, pp 87−98
12. Harzmann R, Weckermann D (1991) Lokale Mikrowellen-Hyperthermie bei der benignen Prostatahyperplasie. Dtsch Ärztebl 88:859−864
13. Harzmann R, Weckermann D (1991) Lokale Hyperthermie bei Prostataerkrankungen? Aktuel Urol 22:10−14
14. Hashimoto T, Hisazumi H, Nakajima K, Matsubara F (1991) Studies on endocrine changes induced by 8 MHz local radiofrequency hyperthermia in patients with bladder cancer. Int J Hyperthermia 7:551−557
15. Hisazumi H, Nakajima K (1988) Eight-MHz RF hyperthermia for urological malignancies. Jpn J Cancer Chemother 15:1382−1386
16. Kaver J, Ware JL, Koontz WW (1989) The effect of hyperthermia on human prostatic carcinoma cell lines: evaluation in vitro. J Urol 141:1025−1027
17. Kaver J; Koontz WJ, Wilson JD, Guice JM, Ware JL (1991) The effect of radiation therapy and hyperthermia on a human prostatic carcinoma cell line in athymic nude mice. J Urol 145:654−656
18. Leib Z, Lev A, Goren E, Servadio C (1991) Observations on the influence of cyproterone acetate on the sonographic image of the benign prostate in patients treated with local hyperthermia. World J Urol 9:19−21
19. Lindner A, Siegel YJ, Saranea R, Korzak D, Matzkin H, Braf Z (1990) Complications in hyperthemia treatment of benign prostatic hyperplasia. J Urol 144:1390−1391
20. Meshorer A (1990) Treatment of benign prostatic hypertrophy using the Thermex II: canine studies. Eur Urol 18
21. Nishimura Y, Hiraoka M, Jo S, Akuta K, Nagata Y, Takahaski M, Abe M (1989) Radiofrequency (RF) capacitive hyperthermia combined with radiotherapy in the treatment of abdominal and pelvic deep-seated tumors. Radiother Oncol 16:139−149
22. Rigatti P, Trabucchi E, Colombo R, Guazzoni G, Maffezzini M, Consonni P, Montorsi F (1989) Hyperthermia induced histological and ultrastructural changes of the prostate. J Urol 141
23. Sapozink MD, Boyd SD, Astrahan MA, Jozsef G, Petrovich Z (1990) Transurethral hyperthermia for benign prostatic hyperplasia: preliminary clinical results, J Urol 143:944−950
24. Schulman CC, Vandenbossche M (1992) Hyperthermia of the prostate as an alternative treatment for benign prostatic hyperplasia. In: Williams D (ed) Rob and Smith's operative surgery: urology, 5th ed. Butterworths, London (in press)
25. Servadio C, Braf Z, Siegel Y, Leib Z, Saranga R, Lindner A (1990) Local thermotherapy of the benign prostate. Eur Urol 18:169−173
26. Strohmaier WL, Bichler K-H, Flüchter SH, Wilbert DM (1990) Local microwave hyperthermia of benign prostatic hyperplasia. J Urol 144:913−917
27. Yerushalmi A, Fishelovitz Y, Singer D, Reiner I, Arielly A, Abramovici Y, Catsenelson R, Levy E, Shani A (1985) Localized deep microwave hyperthermia in the treatment of poor operative risk patients with benign prostatic hyperplasia. J Urol 133:873−876

Transrectal Hyperthermia in Benign Prostatic Hyperplasia

P. Van Erps and L. J. Denis[1]

Introduction

Hyperthermia, or abnormally high temperature of the human body or parts of it, has been induced artifically to promote healing since ancient times. The antitumor effect of heat was first reported by Busch in 1866, who noted that a histologically confirmed sarcoma regressed in a patient following an attack of high fever caused by erysipelas. It has been clearly established that controlled elevation of temperature to the hyperthermic range of 42°−45°C can selectively damage malignant tissue, while leaving surrounding normal tissue unharmed. Although there are many theories concerning the sensitivity of tumor cells to heating, the most important factor is probably defective heat dissipation by neoplastic tissue that occurs as a result of poor blood supply and decreased vasodilation capacity of the neovascular bed in response to thermal load. Tissue overheating causes extensive local cellular damage [1]. A synergistic effect has been shown between hyperthermia and radiotherapy as well as between hyperthermia and several chemotherapeutic agents [2, 3].

Today, many centers around the world use hyperthermia to treat various malignancies. A review of results of clinical studies from several countries demonstrates that hyperthermia is effective in the treatment of cancer, is limited when used alone, and when combined with radiation therapy, is more effective than radiation alone. Nevertheless, the lack of noninvasive thermometric procedures and the technological problems of heat application to deep-seated tumors limit the widespread clinical implementation of this technique.

In the treatment of prostate cancer and benign prostatic hyperplasia (BPH), clinicians have used entry through the rectum to apply heat locally to the tumor. Studies applying local, deep microwave heat (43°C)

[1] Algemeen Ziekenhuis Middelheim, Lindendreef 1, B-2020 Antwerpen, Belgium

to the prostates of rabbits [4] and dogs [5] have shown that the technique and method of application are safe and effective in these animal models. The first group of patients with prostatic cancer treated with local hyperthermia benefited in regard to lessening of obstructive symptoms and reduction in tumor mass [6]. These results led to the application of local hyperthermia to patients with BPH. Over the past 6 years, several reports, primarily from Israel (where the technique was developed), have advocated the use of hyperthermia in treating BPH [7−12]. Up to 70% improvement in objective symptoms and 90% improvement in subjective symptoms have been reported.

The two marketing pioneers for transrectal heating of the prostate gland are Promeditech (Biodan) and Primus (Tecnomatix Medical). In the Primus system the prostate temperature during treatment is calculated by an algorithm, which avoids the need for catheterization at every treatment. We are currently using the Primus system in our department in a phase II study to evaluate the safety and efficacy in BPH.

Patients and Methods

A total of 138 men aged 47−89 years with symptomatic benign prostatic obstruction have undergone transrectal hyperthermia since January 1989. The criteria for entry into the study were: (a) age over 50 years, (b) prostate (adenoma) weighing 20−60 g, (c) high symptom score, (d) max Q of 5−15 ml/s and (e) residual volume under 200 ml.

Exclusion criteria were:

− significant urinary tract anomalies (large diverticula, neurogenic bladder hydronephrosis) serum creatinine over 2.0 mg%
− confirmed malignancy of the prostate,
− significant rectal pathology,
− acute prostatitis,
− urinary tract infection,
− bladder neck fibrosis, and
− large median lobe.

All patients had symptoms for at least 6 months, and close analysis of the symptom status was carried out using a modified Boyarski scoring system (Table 1). Patients underwent an extensive preliminary investigation in our prostate clinic, and these examinations were repeated every 3 months during the first year of follow-up and every 6 months thereafter. The examinations included:

Table 1. Symptom score scale

	Scale			
	0	1	2	3
Frequency	Normal (1–4×)	Mild (5–7×)	Moderate (8–12×)	Severe (13×)
Nocturia	0	1	2–3×	>3
Quality of stream	Good	Satisfactory	Weak	Poor
Urgency	No	Slight	Mild	Severe
Hesitancy	No	Slight	Mild	Severe

- physical examination (digital palpation);
- uroflow (voided volume >150 ml) – total time, peak flow rate, average flow;
- blood (prostate-specific antigen, PSA; prostatic acid phosphatase), ureum; creatinine) and urine;
- prostate volume by transrectal ultrasound;
- residual urine by transabdominal ultrasound;
- adverse effects; and
- questionnaire.

Urinary performance was assessed by the peak and average urinary flow rates, measured on several occasions, and residual volume measured by postmicturition ultrasound examination. Other causes of outflow obstruction were excluded by careful urodynamic investigation and cystoscopy. Transrectal sonographic images (Bruel and Kjaer, Aloka) were obtained to ascertain the benign nature of the prostate and to assess the size of the gland. All patients were free of urinary infection at the time of the treatment. In a questionnaire the patients were asked to evaluate their urinary status after treatment on a seven-point scale with 4 points for no change, 1 point for excellent as compared to pretreatment, and 7 points for a much worse situation after treatment.

Hyperthermia Unit Description

All patients were treated with the Primus transrectal hyperthermia system (developed by Tecnomatix Medical, Antwerp, Belgium) comprising the following components:

- A power generator, with an output power of 0–40 W and operating at frequencies of 915 MHz.
- A closed loop water cooling unit for maintaining the rectal temperature at the desired level (temperature range 8°–24°C).
- The unit is controlled by an IBM computer with software for automatic and manual operation, analog and digital temperature monitoring and display of treatment parameters, and data collection. A computer algorithm calculates the prostate temperature, which avoids invasive catheterization in every treatment.
- The finger-shaped transrectal applicator contains the microwave antenna, cooling channels, and three thermocouples.

The applicator is composed of Teflon, 20 mm in outside diameter, with a rounded distal end. Spiral coils circulate cold water just inside the applicator surface to cool the rectal mucosa.

Microwave power is emitted from a 915-MHz dipole antenna embedded centrally in the applicator with a 180°C reflector in the posterior half.

Three thermocouples are affixed to the active directional wall of the applicator. The copper constantan couples are totally sheeted with Teflon.

Treatment Procedure

The treatment procedure was as follows:

- Outpatient basis
- No sedation or anesthesia
- Cover applicator with rubber condom, gel for comfort
- Introduce applicator, directed to prostate mass
- Thermometry – Temperatures are monitored during treatment on the screen:
  Interface rectal mucosa and antenna
  Prostate calculated temperature by computer algorithm
  Treatment schedule
  Treatment time: 60 min
  Number of treatments per week: two
  Total number of sessions: ten
  Prostate calculated temperature: 43 °C

All treatments were conducted on an outpatient basis without sedation or anesthesia. After covering with a rubber condom, the applicator was inserted in the rectum to the depth previously determined by ultrasound, so that the dipole antenna faces the maximal dimensions of the prostate. The treatment was started, and the power was raised step by step following a fixed heat-up program. Further on, the power was kept on automatic mode, and the cooling was adjusted so that the temperature reading on the antenna did not exceed 39°C, and a prostate calculated temperature of 43°C was obtained in all treatments. All temperature data were recorded on the computer every 15s. The hyperthermia treatment was given in ten sessions of 60min each, twice weekly over 5 weeks.

Results

Overall, transrectal hyperthermia was easy to perform and was well tolerated by our patients. No anesthesia or sedation was required during any of·the treatments. No complications occurred during the treatment, and in only tqo patients was treatment discontinued as a result of rectal pain. Most patients had a sensation of local heating within the pelvis. Bladder spasms with urgent voiding were experienced by a few patients. The subjective response in 136 patients at 3 months after the treatment was as follows. A score of 1 or 2 was given by 88 patients (65%) on the seven-point scale, which means that they felt excellent or very much improved after the treatment. Another 20 patients (14%) felt better, 26 patients (19%) experienced no change, while only 2 patients felt worse after treatment. Analysis of the Boyarski symptom score in the 88 patients who gave a 1 or 2 score shows a decrease in the mean score pretreatment of 8.46 to a mean score posttreatment of 3.61. The mean values of the symptoms for the whole group of patients, with standard deviations pre- and posttreatment, are given in Table 2.

In the objective response of 136 patients at 3 months we consider an improvement in maximum flow (Q_{max}) of 50% or more for the same voided volume as an objective response. Thirty-three patients (24%) showed this improvement of flow measured on several occasions, with

Table 2. Mean values of symptoms ($\pm$ SD)

	Pretreatment	Posttreatment
Nocturia	1.9 ± 0.85	1.3 ± 0.8
Frequency	1.7 ± 0.82	$1 \ \ \pm 0.7$
Resistance	1.5 ± 0.89	0.8 ± 0.8
Urgency	1.6 ± 0.98	0.7 ± 0.8
Impairment	$2 \ \ \pm 0.6$	$1 \ \ \pm 0.88$
Total Score	8.7 ± 2.3	4.9 ± 2.8

Table 3. Results at 1-year follow-up ($n = 60$)

	n	%
Subjective criteria		
Responders ($n = 39$)		
Status quo	28	72
Death	2	5
TURP	5	12
No follow-up	4	10
Nonresponders ($n = 21$)		
Status quo	8	38
Transurethral HPT	1	4
TURP	9	42
No follow-up	3	14
Objective criteria		
Responders ($n = 19$)		
Status quo	15	79
Death	1	5
TURP	2	10
No follow-up	1	5
Nonresponders ($n = 41$)		
Status quo	21	51
Death	1	2
TURP	12	29
Transurethral HPT	1	2
No follow-up	6	15

an increase from 8.3 to 15.0. In the 103 showing no objective response the increase was from 9.2 to 9.7. For the whole group, Q_{max} changed from 9 ml/s before to 10.8 ml/s after treatment (not statistically significant). The size of the prostate as measured by transrectal sonographic images did not change after treatment. During treatment a temporary rise in PSA was possible to a threefold level, but all specific antigen values returned to the pretreatment level after 1 month.

The outcome at 1-year follow-up is summarized in Table 3. Of the 39 subjective responders, 28 (72%) were still happy 1 year after finishing the treatment while only 5 patients (12%) of the responders were treated by TURP. Fifteen (79%) of the 19 objective responders maintained status quo 1 year after finishing the treatment while only 2 patients (10%) of this group were treated by TURP.

Discussion

The classic treatment of BPH with obstruction is TURP because of the high success rates and low morbidity in the hands of experienced urologists [13]. Although TURP is widely percieved by urologists as a successful operation, there is some morbidity and a small failure rate [14, 15]. Many men suffering with symptoms of early prostatic obstruction and well-preserved detrusor function are not considered candidates for operative treatment but might benefit from a minimally invasive treatment. Other groups of patients who are suitable for such treatment are those in whom preservation of the antegrade ejaculation is important and those with a neurologic problem such as Parkinson's disease, where the outcome of TURP is less satisfactory.

Balloon dilation of the prostate does not meet the criteria of a minimally invasive technique since spinal anesthesia and hospital admission are required [16]. Stents in the prostatic urethra can be placed with topical anesthesia alone, but concern remains about the long-term risks of prosthetic materials within the urinary tract [17]. The great hope of finding a medication that replaces prostatic surgery still seems to be some way off; in selected patients selective alpha-blockers may produce symptomatic and objective improvement [18]. The place of finasteride (a 5-alpha-reductase inhibitor) has yet to be established, but it is obvious that a lifetime commitment to treatment is required because of the rapid regrowth of the prostate once normal testosterone stimulation resumes [19]. Treatment of benign prostatic obstruction by transrectal microwave therapy has been reported as having a success rate of 50% in rendering patients catheter free, with 40% still voiding at 1 year [20]. Large increases in flow rate in patients treated by transrectal hyperthermia were initially reported by Lindner and associates in 1987 [21]. Subsequently the number of patients showing objective improvement has been observed to be 42%, while 50% of patients reported subjective improvement at 3 months [22].

In our series we found a higher subjective improvement at 65%, and a lower objective improvement at 24%, but the objective evaluation criteria are difficult to compare. Taking into account the spontaneous fluctuations in the clinical course of BPH [23], the objective improvement in our series was not impressive at all. Our study does not provide controls, and any conclusions drawn must consider the widely recognized placebo effect observed in both subjective and objective variables measured in many BPH studies. However, the symptom response has been excellent in two-thirds of our patients, and patients feel that they can pass urine more freely than before even when there is little evidence of objective improvement.

The mechanism of action of transrectal hyperthermia is still unclear. Transrectal hyperthermia probably produces a relaxation of the prostatic smooth muscle, and the similarity between our results and the results of alpha-blockade favor this theory, but we accept that this has yet to be proved.

Two-thirds of our patients with symptomatic BPH benefited from the procedure, which is free of any clinical adverse effects, but placebo-controlled studies and long-term follow-up are needed to clearly establish the role of this new modality in the treatment of BPH.

References

1. Song CW (1978) Effects of hyperthermia on vascular functions of normal tissues and experimental tumors. J N C I 60:711–713
2. Robinson JE, Wizenberg MJ (1974) Thermal sensitivity and the effect of elevated temperatures on the radiation sensitivity of Chinese hamster cells. Acta Radiol Ther 13:241–248
3. Marmor JB (1979) Interactions of hyperthermia and chemotherapy in animals. Cancer Res 39:2269–2276
4. Yerushalmi A, Shpirer Z, Hod I, Gottesfeld F, Bass DD (1982) Normal tissue response to localized deep microwave hyperthermia in the rabbit's prostate: a preclinical study. Int J Radiat Oncol Biol Phys 9:77–82
5. Leib Z, Rothem A, Lev A, Servadio C (1986) Histopathological observations in the canine prostate treated by local microwave hyperthermia. Prostate 8:93–102
6. Yerushalmi A, Servadio C, Leib Z, Fishelovitz Y, Rokowsky E, Stein JA (1982) Local hyperthermia for treatment of carcinoma of the prostate: a preliminary report. Prostate 6:623
7. Yerushalmi A, Fishelovitz Y, Singer D, Reiner I, Arielly J, Abramovici Y et al. (1985) Localized deep microwave hyperthermia in the treatment of poor operative risk patients with benign prostatic hyperplasia. J Urol 133:873–876
8. Servadio C, Leib Z, Lev A (1986) Further observations on the use of local hyperthermia for the treatment of diseases of the prostate in man. Eur Urol 12:38–40
9. Servadio C, Leib Z, Lev A (1987) Diseases of prostate treated by local microwave hyperthermia. Urology 30:97–99
10. Servadio C, Lev A, Leib Z (1988) Local hyperthermia for the treatment of diseases of the prostate. J Urol 139:484A
11. Lindner A, Golomb J, Siegel Y, Lev A (1987) Local hyperthermia of the prostate gland for the treatment of benign prostatic hypertrophy and urinary retention: a preliminary report. Br J Urol 60:567–571
12. Yerushalmi A (1988) Localized, non-invasive deep microwave hyperthermia for the treatment of prostatic tumors: the first 5 years. Recent Results Cancer Res 107:141–146
13. Blandy J (1986) The history and current problems of benign prostatic obstruction in the prostate. Butterworths, London, pp 12–22
14. Mebust WK, Holtgrewe HL, Cockett ATK et al. (1989) Transurethral prostatectomy: immediate and postoperative complications: a cooperative study of 13 participating institutions evaluating 3885 patients. J Urol 141:243

15. Fowler FJ, Wennberg JE, Timothy RP et al. (1988) Symptom status and quality of life following prostatectomy. JAMA 259:3018
16. Dowd JB, Smith JJ (1990) Balloon dilation of the prostate. Urol Clin North Am 17:671
17. Chapple C, Milroy EJ, Rickards D (1990) Permanently implanted urethral stent for prostatic obstruction in the unfit patient: preliminary report. Br J Urol 66:58
18. Caine M (1990) Alpha-adrenergic blockers for the treatment of benign prostatic hyperplasia. Urol Clin North Am 17:641
19. McConnell JD (1990) Androgen blockade in the treatment of benign prostic hyperplasia. Urol Clin North Am 17:661
20. Lindner A, Braf Z, Lev A et al. (1990) Local hyperthermia of the prostate gland for the treatment of benign prostatic hypertrophy and urinary retention. Br J Urol 65:201
21. Lindner A, Golomb J, Siegal Y, Lev A (1987) Local hyperthermia of the prostate gland for the treatment of benign prostatic hypertrophy and urinary retention: a preliminary report. Br J Urol 60:567
22. Saranga R, Matzkin H, Braf Z (1990) Local microwave hyperthermia of the prostate gland in the treatment of benign prostic hypertrophy. Br J Urol 65:349
23. Ball AJ, Feneley RCL, Abrams PH (1981) The natural history of untreated „prostatism". Br J Urol 53:613

Transurethral Microwave Thermotherapy of the Prostate: Principles and Early Clinical Results*

M. Devonec, M. Cathaud, J. P. Fendler, G. Bringeon, T. Dujardin, and P. Perrin[1]

The goal of this study was to treat urinary obstruction related to benign prostatic hypertrophy by destroying prostatic tissue deep within the prostate with microwaves, while preserving urethral tissue and avoiding localized pain. The idea was to treat both the dynamic and the mechanical components of prostatic obstruction. The microwaves are delivered transurethrally by means of a flexible applicator during a single session of short duration.

Principles of Transurethral Microwave Thermotherapy

To destroy intraprostatic tissue to a depth of 10−15 mm from the urethra, the power required would raise the urethral temperature to 75°−80°C. At this power and these temperatures, the tissue effect is characterized by necrosis and subsequent sloughing of the dead tissue (Fig. 1). Transurethral hyperthermia (i.e., tissue heating in the range of 42°−44°C) has a limiting factor, namely the occurrence of pain as soon as the urethral temperature reaches 46°C or beyond. This local pain and burning effect prevents the use of higher power in humans [1−4]. Higher power appears to be the only way, however, to induce a deeper effect in the prostate other than the superficial burning of the urethra (Fig. 2). To decrease the urethral temperature and avoid the formation of an intraprostatic cavity, we introduced the principle of urethral cooling (Fig. 3a). Microwave heating is the phenomenon of radiation penetrating tissue at depth. This radiative principle differs from the principle of cooling, which is based on conductivity, and which has a limited action. The result of the combination of these two princi-

[1] Antiquaille Hospital, Department of Urology, Claude Bernard University, 1, rue de l'Antiquaille, F-69321 Lyon Cedex 05, France

* This study was supported in part by a grant from Claude Bernard University, Prix Antonin Poncet.

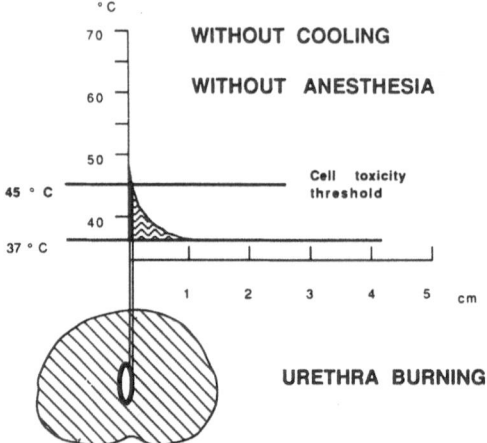

Fig. 1. Theoretical effect of transurethral microwave heating without cooling but under general anesthesia (*x axis,* distance in centimeters from the microwave antenna; *y axis,* temperature in degrees centigrade). The prostatic area with a temperature above 45°C *(dark)* is destroyed and replaced by a cavity

ples, radiative heating and conductive cooling, is a temperature curve (Fig. 3b) with a step ascending slope and a progressive descending slope. As long as the tissue temperature remains below the cell's toxicity threshold, no histological effect is noticed (Fig. 3c). Tissue destruction begins when the ascending slope of the curve goes beyond this toxicity threshold, and it continues as long as the tissue temperature remains above 45°C for at least 30 min. Tissue destruction does not

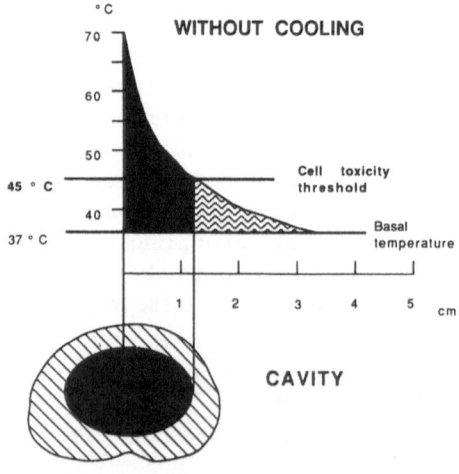

Fig. 2. Theoretical effect of transurethral microwave heating without cooling without anesthesia: power output is rapidly limited by urethral pain and results in a superficial burning of the urethra

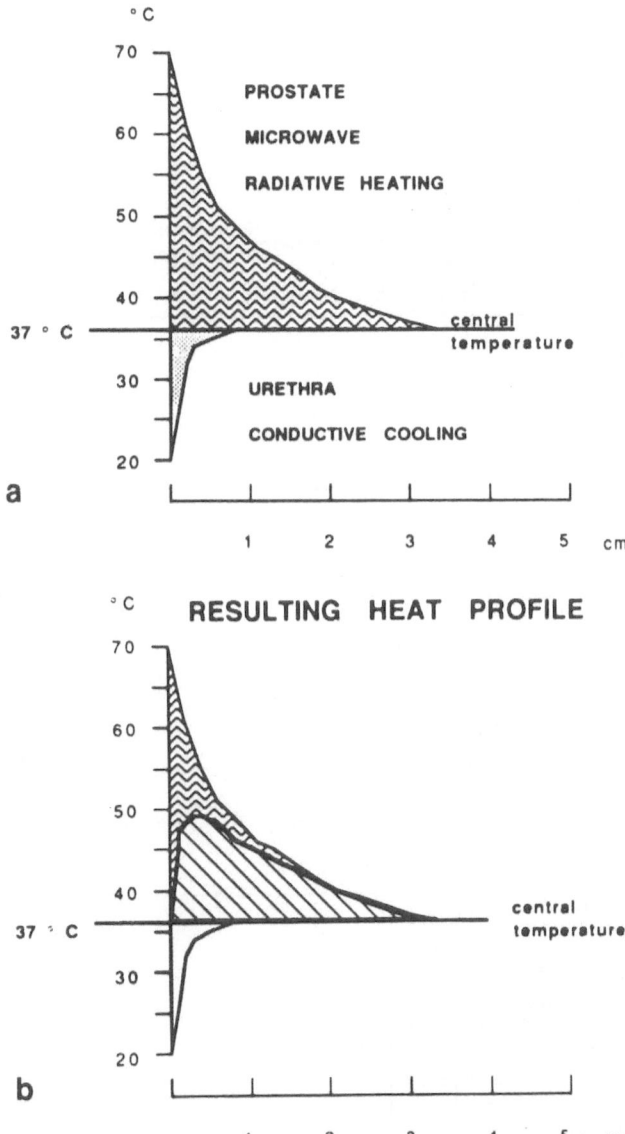

Fig. 3a, b. Transurethral microwave therapy concept (*x axis,* distance in centimeter from the antenna in the urethra; *y axis,* temperature in degrees centigrade). **a** The microwave heating pattern shows that the energy needed to induce deep tissue necrosis would raise the temperature to 70°–80°C in the urethra. Cooling of the urethra was introduced to maintain the urethral temperature at a tolerable level without general anesthesia. **b** The combination of deep radiative heating and superficial conductive cooling leads to an asymmetrical temperature profile, with a steep ascending slope and a progressive descending slope.

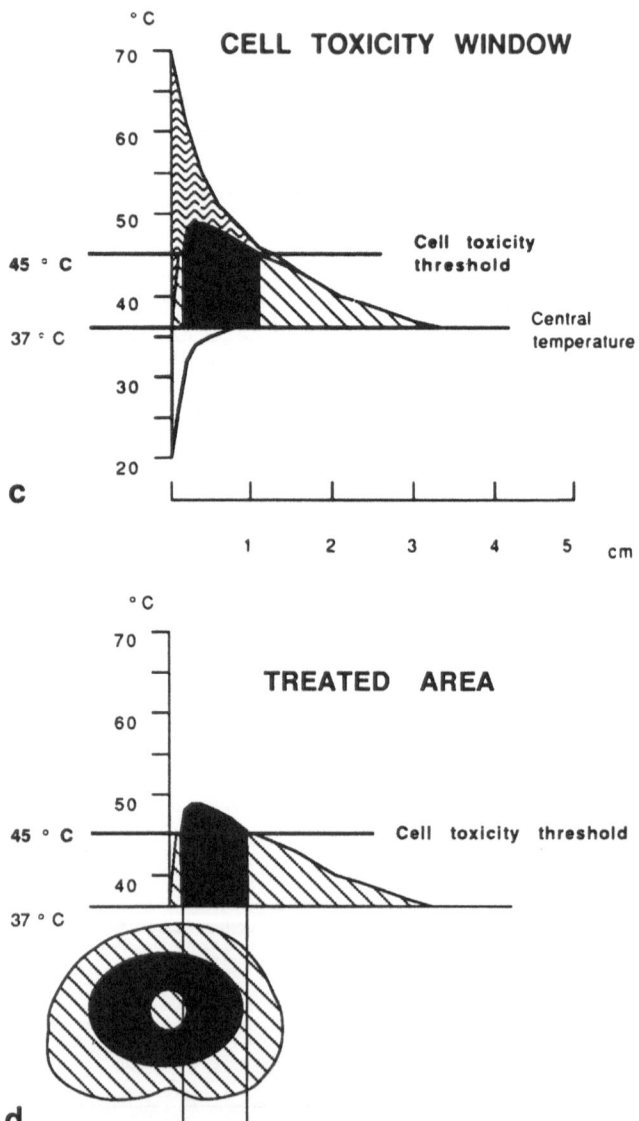

Fig. 3c, d. Transurethral microwave therapy concept (continued). **c** Since the cell toxicity threshold is 45°C for benign prostatic tissue, periurethral tissue is preserved as long as the temperature stays below the therapeutic threshold, i.e., lower than 45°C. Tissue destruction *(area in dark)* is observed as soon as the ascending slope crosses the therapeutic threshold and is maintained until the descending slope crosses it. **d** Theoretical application of the transurethral microwave therapy concept to the prostate. The center of the gland is protected and surrounded by a crown of treated prostatic tissue *(dark)*

occur when the tissue temperature is below 45°C. Consequently, the integration of a cooling system permits the preservation of the urethra and the periurethral mucosa, with the formation of a necrotic tissue area up to a distance of 17 mm from the urethra in some cases (Fig. 3d). The cooling allows urethral temperature to be maintained below the pain level threshold. By preserving the urethra, retrograde ejaculation is avoided.

These results obtained in dogs with this new principle allowed us to start a preclinical trial in a selected group of patients in October 1989, with the agreement of our Ethical Committee. This preclinical study was undertaken before considering the treatment of patients with symptoms of prostatic obstruction related to benign prostatic hypertrophy.

Preclinical Study

From a histological point of view, benign prostatic hyperplasia (BPH) in men is quite different from glandular hyperplasia in dogs [5, 6]. For this reason, we believed that interstitial thermometry, histological examinations, and illustration of temperature sensations to microwave emission in man were required in this preclinical trial to determine whether we could duplicate our animal study results [7].

Thermokinetic Study

Interstitial thermometry was performed in seven patients under general anesthesia prior to transurethral resection. The increase in tissue temperatures was measured by means of optic fibers inserted within the prostate (two fibers) at a distance of 5–20 mm from the microwave antenna, as well in the interprostatorectal Denonvilliers fascia (one fiber) under ultrasound guidance. The urethral and rectal temperatures were automatically recorded. When the urethral cooling reached a steady state, the microwave emission was started and maintained until the intraprostatic temperature reached at least 45°C.

Results from these trials showed that:

1) the intraprostatic temperature can be raised to a therapeutic level (above 45°C) within 15–20 min.
2) urethral cooling is strong enough to keep urethral temperatures below 40°C, and
3) the rectal wall itself appears to be naturally protected by an excellent blood supply against microwave emission.

This accounts for the superiority of the new transurethral approach versus transrectal heating in the treatment of the prostate by microwave power.

Temperature Sensation

Tolerance to urethral heating was investigated in three volunteers using microwaves at low power one day prior to transurethral resection. Initially, the urethra was cooled and stopped when a steady state was reached. Microwave emission was started without resuming cooling. The emission was stopped as soon as the patient complained of discomfort.

This study showed that cooling the urethra at a speed of $-15\,°C$ per minute was well tolerated as well as heating of the urethra at $+3.5\,°C$ per minute. The maximum temperature which could be tolerated at the level of the urethra for a short period of time was $47\,°C$.

These preclinical trials confirmed that TransUrethral Microwave Thermotherapy (TUMT) can be safely administered, and there is a tissue effect clearly shown in histological examination. Clinical trials were subsequently started in patients with symptomatic prostatic obstruction resulting from BPH using a new microwave device (Prostatron, Technomed international; Fig. 4).

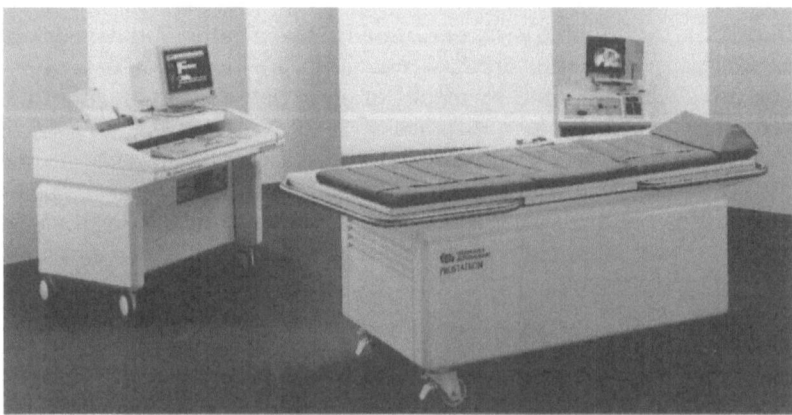

Fig. 4. Prostatron. Treatment module and control module

Results of Early Clinical Trials

Materials and Methods

This study included 37 BPH patients with urinary flow rates of less than 15 ml/s and a voided volume of more than 150 ml [8, 9]. A digital rectal examination and transrectal ultrasonography were performed to rule out the presence of carcinoma.

The treatment was performed on an outpatient basis for all patients. After instillation of anesthetic lubricant in the urethra, the bladder was emptied and the postresidual volume was measured. One hundred milliliters of sterile water were injected into the bladder before the insertion of the urethral catheter containing the microwave antenna. The Foley-type balloon was inflated, and its correct positioning, i.e., balloon in contact with the bladder neck, was checked by ultrasound with the patient in the left lateral decubitus position. The rectal temperature was measured with a mercury thermometer, and the rectal probe, designed for controlling the temperature of the rectal wall, was then inserted and fixed in place.

The patient resumed the supine position and the first phase of the treatment was started. This consisted of cooling the urethra, which rapidly occurred over a few minutes. The microwave emission was then automatically started and increased gradually to a maximum of 55 W, or until a temperature of 42.5 °C in the rectum was reached, whichever came first. When the maximum power level was reached within the preset safety limits, the third phase of the treatment was started by progressively warming the urethra (decreasing the cooling) to increase and widen the field of the treated tissue. Based on our previous work, safety limits were set at 42.5 °C at the level of the rectum and 45 °C in the urethra. When the rectal temperature reached its maximum level, the microwave emission was stopped and resumed at the same level minus 5 W after the measured rectal temperature had decreased by 0.5 °C. When the urethral temperature reached 45 °C, final adjustment was achieved by making use of the two mechanisms available: temporary interruption of microwave emission and/or changes in the cooling system parameters. The microwave emission was at all times monitored automatically by the computer through the assessment of the rectal and urethral temperatures. The total treatment duration was 55 min.

Results

The urethral, rectal, and vesical tolerance was good. in three patients, the physician had to manually decrease the power output to achieve patient comfort. No treatment had to be interrupted due to patient discomfort. The patient symptom score (derived from Boyarsky) was significantly improved at 3 months; in particular, improvement in nocturia was mentioned by a majority of patients. Improvement in peak flow was statistically significant but with a moderate increase; other centers are already obtaining better results in peak flow than ours, using the same device [10]. This difference may reflect patient selection bias in series with small numbers; but more importantly the introduction over time of slight modifications in the treatment regimen lead to an increase in the thermal dose delivered to the last patients of our series when compared to the earlier ones. Postresidual volume decreased significantly although ultrasound measurement via the suprapubic route lacks accuracy. Prostate volume remained the same, probably due to the width of the remaining nontreated peripheral and transition zones, which prevents the prostate from shrinking, whereas the 2- to 5-mm preserved urethral tissue retracts from the center of the gland towords the periphery as a consequence of the healing of the treated prostatic tissue and results in urethra decompression. PSA was significantly increased by day 7 and related to acinar cell damage by heat. Experience will tell whether PSA or another serum marker might be used in the future as a predictor of prostatic tissue response to heat. Due to the variation in prostate histology, patient hydration, and vascularization, tissue response to heat may be very different from one patient to another despite the similarity of prostatic volume. These results were obtained with intraprostatic temperatures above 45°C. The range of temperatures used for TransUrethral Microwave Thermotherapy of the prostate are significantly higher than those used for prostatic hyperthermia (42−44°C). According to our histological results, it appears that the cell toxicity threshold for benign adenomatous tissue is above 45°C, and that temperatures need to reach between 45−55°C for significant results to be obtained. No complications were observed at the level of the rectum, sphincter, or ureteral meatus. Following treatment, seven patients had urinary retention and required an indwelling catheter for one week. Four of these seven patients are now voiding satisfactorily. The other three patients were eventually resected because of poor bladder emptying.

These early clinical results show that a single session of microwave Thermotherapy performed on an outpatient basis can induce a significant improvement in objective and subjective urinary obstructive symptoms with an acceptable tolerance and in the absence of any significant complications. There has been no retreatment needed for any of the 34 patients (excluding the three patients who required resection) who were initially treated. Long-term follow-up of these patients (1 year) continues and will be reported in subsequent publications.

Acknowledgements. The authors are indebted to J. Finzi for excellent technical assistance and to Prof. J. L. Peix, head of the experimental surgery laboratory where animal studies were conducted.

References

1. Astrahan MA, Sapozink MD, Cohen D, Luxton GL, Kampp TD, Boyd S, Petrovich Z (1989) Microwave applicator for transurethral hyperthermia of benign prostatic hyperplasia. Int J Hyperthermia 5:283
2. Sapozink MD, Boyd SD, Astrahan MA, Jozsef G, Petrovich Z (1990) Transurethral hyperthermia for benign prostatic hyperplasia: preliminary clinical results. J Urol 143:944–950
3. Baert L, Ameye P, Willemein P, D'Hallewin MA (1990) Transurethral hyperthermia for BPH and prostatodymia: preliminary clinical and pathological results. J Urol 143:413A
4. Schulman CC, van den Bosche M (1990) Hyperthermia with the Thermex II for benign prostatic hypertrophy. Proceedings of the 9th IXth congress of the European Association of Urology, June 1990, Amsterdam, p 265
5. Devonec M, Carter S, Perrin P (1989) Prostatic obstruction – a new system. Proceedings of the British Association of Urological Surgeons, June 1989, St. Helier, Jersey, p 98
6. Devonec M, Cathaud M, Mouriquand P, Maquet JH, Oukheira H, Dutrieux-Berger N, Perrin P (1989) Effects of transurethral microwave heating on the canine prostate. Proceedings of the 7th world congress on endourology and Extracorporeal Shock Wave Lithotripsy, November 1989, Kyoto, p 73
7. Devonec M, Cathaud M, Carter S, Dutrieux-Berger N, Perrin P (1990) Transurethral microwave application: temperature sensation and thermokinetics of the human prostate. J Urol 143:414A
8. Devonec M, Cathaud M, Carter S, Dutrieux-Berger N, Perrin P (1990) The effects of transurethral microwave thermotherapy (TUMT) in patients with benign prostatic hypertrophy. In: Proceedings of the 9th congress of the European Association of Urology, June 1990, Amsterdam, p 265
9. Devonec M, Cathaud M, Carter S, Dutrieux-Berger N, Perrin P (1990) Histological and clinical effects of transurethral microwave therapy in patients with benign prostatic hypertrophy. 42rd congress of the Deutsche Gesellschaft für Urologie, September 1990, Hamburg
10. Carter S, Patel A, Perrin P, Devonec M (1990) Objective clinical results of transurethral microwave thermotherapy for benign prostatic obstruction. J Endourol 4 [Suppl I]:134

Medical Treatment

Is Pharmacotherapy for Benign Prostatic Hyperplasia an Alternative?

C. R. Chapple[1]

Introduction

Benign prostatic hyperplasia (BPH) is probably the commonest benign human neoplasm. Histologically identifiable hyperplastic changes in the prostate are present in approximately 50% of men at the age of 60 and in nearly 100% of men by 80 years [39]. Although the histological prevalence of a disease cannot be equated with its associated clinical picture, it has been reported that three-quarters of men over the age of 50 will suffer symptoms suggestive of BPH. Furthermore, it is estimated that the prevalence of significant BPH, defined as an enlargement of the prostate gland greater than 15 ml/s in the presence of symptoms and/or a urinary flow rate under 15 ml/s; and without evidence of malignancy, was 253/1000 in a sample of 705 men aged 40–79 registered with a group general practice in Scotland [27]. In the United States Glynn et al. [32] calculated the chance of a 40-year-old man subsequently requiring a prostatectomy as 29%.

Recent reports of the significant morbidity and mortality which may be associated with transurethral prostatectomy, coupled with re-operation rates of 8.9%–9.7% at 5 years, rising to 12%–15.5% at 8 years [60] and increased public awareness of alternative non-surgical or minimally invasive treatment options have all contributed to the increased interest in the use of pharmacotherapy for the treatment of BPH. Indeed, out of the 350000 men diagnosed annually in the United Kingdom as having clinical problems attributable to BPH, only 10% undergo surgery. It must be remembered that although the symptom complex in BPH results from urethral obstruction, many patients are in fact most troubled by the „irritative" symptoms associated with the secondary detrusor instability, which occurs in up to 75% of patients [3].

---

[1] The Royal Hallamshire Hospital, Department of Urology, Glossop Road, Sheffield S10 2JF, UK

Table 1. Natural history of untreated BPH, based on 4 studies[a]

Response	Subjective	Objective
Improvement	38% ± 4%	22%
No change	16% ± 9%	16%
Worsening	45% ± 7%	63%

[a] A total of 282 patients were followed up for 2.6−5 years; data from [5, 6a, 21a, 22] (from [39]).

Before reviewing the results of drug therapy it must be realised that the natural history course of untreated prostatic obstruction is very variable [5, 14, 22], with slow progression, no change or even improvement of patients' symptoms on conservative management alone (Table 1). Improvements after any therapy investigated in the short term may not therefore relate to the treatment but many rather reflect the natural history of the disease process itself. The patient should be properly investigated prior to the instigation of pharmacotherapy, not only so that a satisfactory appraisal of efficacy can be obtained, but also so that prostatic malignancy and other complications of prostatic obstruction or other coexisting disease such as bladder cancer are not missed. Furthermore, one must reconcile oneself to the absence of the tissue diagnosis automatically obtained following prostatectomy, with the associated likelihood of missing up to one-fifth of patients with focal carcinoma [20].

BPH is an important cause of bladder outflow obstruction. Both a *static* factor, due to the mechanical compression exerted by the increased bulk of prostate in BPH, and fluctuating − so-called *Dynamic* − influences, resulting from alterations in the neural control of prostatic muscle control are important. Pharmacotherapy can potentially be effective by *reducing* prostatic size acting via a hormonal mechanism of action or *relaxing* prostatic muscle by blockade of sympathetic adrenergic nerves. The assessment of such therapy must be carried out using double-blinded placebo-controlled studies not only because of the random fluctuations in symptoms which occur in patients with symptomatic BPH, but also because of the significant placebo effects in controlled trials reported to date (Table 2).

Hormonal Therapy

Whilst the precise mechanisms underlying the development of pathogenesis of BPH are poorly understood, it seems clear that hor-

Table 2. Placebo effect of drugs on BPH, based on 12 studies[a]

Response	Subjective	Objective
Improvement	42% ± 5%	24% ± 6%
No change	46% ± 6%	58% ± 11%
Worsening	12% ± 2%	19% ± 7%

[a] A total of 260 patients were followed up for 0.6−6 months; data from [1, 2, 8, 10, 12, 14, 22a, 29, 32, 44, 59, 59a] (from [39]).

monal factors are important in its pathogenesis. John Hunter [37] was the first to document clearly the relationship between the testes and prostatic growth, when in 1786 he noted that castration of animals produced a reduction in prostatic size and function. The earliest hormonal therapy used in man can be attributed to the treatment of BPH by surgical castration [9, 70]. In a study of 111 cases treated by castration, White noted a marked reduction in prostatic size. Of 61 patients who had undergone castration, who were reported by Cabot the following year, urinary retention disappeared in 27, and the majority of patients were markedly improved. Moore [54] reported the most comprehensive study in support of this relationship between the testes and the pathogenesis of BPH to date. In this study, absent testicular function (castration or hypopituitarism) prior to the age of 40 years prevented the occurrence of BPH or prostate cancer in men who lived into the BPH age group (over 55 years). Further evidence in support of these observations is provided by a study of the Russian Skoptzys sect, which practices ritual castration of men at the age of 35 years, and who appreared to be spared the development of BPH [71].

Although there are no significant differences in androgen levels in age-matched men with and without BPH [6], it seems likely that androgens provide a hormonal milieu that is essential to the development of BPH. A number of theories exist as to the mechanism of development of BPH [30], further consideration of which is beyond the scope of this article.

Despite the efficacy of castration the advent of endoscopic resection of the prostate resulted in a diminution in interest. Geller and associates were amongst the first to rekindle interest in this field with study of the progestational agent megesterol acetate in an uncontrolled study reported in 1965 [28]. Subsequently a number of drugs have been used competitively to antagonise the trophic effects of androgens on the prostate, using drugs acting at various levels on the neuro-endocrine axis (Fig. 1). A representative selection of these studies is summarised in Table 3.

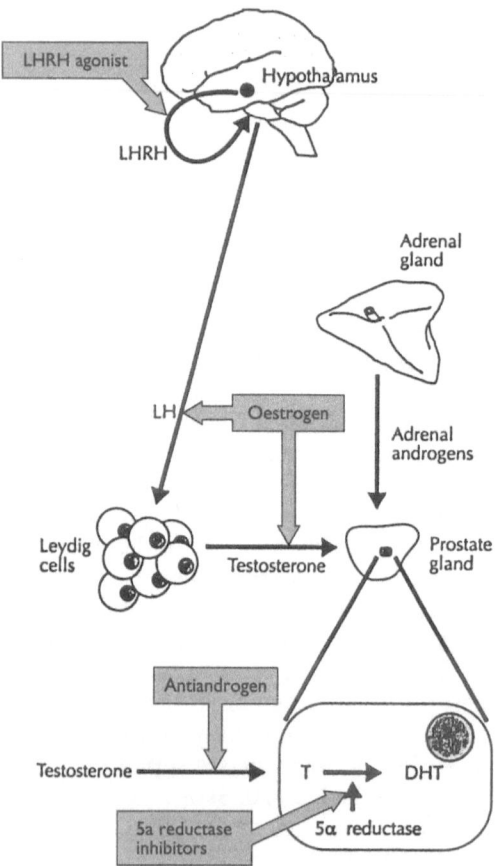

Fig. 1. Control of androgen production by the hypothalamic-pituitary system. Sites of action of pharmalogical agents that reduce prostate bulk

It is evident from these data that hormonal therapy is effective, but noticeably less so than surgery. It is becoming increasingly clear that certain subgroups of patients are more likely to respond to hormonal blockade than others. It may be that the reason for this lies with the underlying prostatic histology, in particular the relative proportions of epithelial and stromal components. Indeed, the observation by Huggins and Stevens [36], when reviewed in retrospect, provides some interesting insight into the potential limitations of anti-androgen therapy. In three patients with BPH following castration, significant epithelial atrophy did not occur until 90 days after hormonal withdrawal, and there was little change in the stroma. Recent evidence has

Table 3. Representative clinical studies evaluating androgen deprivation for BPH (from [46a])

Reference	Drug	Randomised placebo-controlled	n	Weeks of study	Change in prostate size	Change in urinary flow rate	Improved symptom score	Conclusion
Scott et al. (1969) [62]	Cyproterone acetate	No	13	Variable	Not measured	Increase	Not measured	Effective
Caine et al. (1975) [10]	Flutamide	Yes	30	12	Not measured	Significant increase	Not measured	Effective
Geller et al. (1979) [29]	Megesterol acetate	Yes	61	20	Not measured	Significant increase	Not measured	Effective
Donkervoort et al. (1975) [24]	Megesterol acetate	No	36	16	Not measured	Increase	Yes	Inconclusive
Meiraz et al. (1977) [52]	17-Hydroxy progesterone	No	39	14	No significant change	Not measured	No significant change	Ineffective
Peters et al. (1987) [57]	Nafarelin acetate	No	8	27	24% decrease in size	Increase in some patients	Improved in 6/9 patients	Inconclusive
Matzkin et al. (1991) [51]	Triptorelin	No	17 10	24 48	27% decrease in size	Increase in some patients	Improved in 10/17 patients	Limited role

been put forward which suggests that serum prostatic-specific antigen (PSA) may be helpful in predicting response to hormonal therapy [49, 51]. Serum PSA appears to reflect the ratio between epithelial and stromal components within the prostate; although PSA is positively correlated with prostatic volume, PSA is also correlated with the degree of prostatic epithelial hyperplasia. The patients who respond best to this therapy are those with a higher serum PSA and a smaller prostatic volume.

A major disadvantage of all these therapies has been the high incidence of unwanted side effects, many of which can be attributed to a reduction in systemic circulating androgens (loss of libido, impotence). The development of specific androgen blockade within the prostate by inhibition of the enzyme 5α-reductase, thereby preventing the conversion of testosterone to the active derivative dihydrotestosterone (DHT), was potentially a major advance. This provides a specific hormonal effect without reducing circulating extra-prostatic androgen and thereby avoids unwanted side effects consequent upon androgen withdrawal. The initial clinical studies have yielded disappointing results, with improvements in mean urinary flow rate of only a few milliliters per second, despite significant reductions in prostatic size and quantitative symptom scoring [64]. Really, this is not surprising since the results would not be expected to be superior to those to be obtained following castration. From the preliminary results which are available, there do appear to be significant inter-subject variations in response within the studies similar to those noted with previous studies of hormonal therapy for BPH, no doubt for similar reasons.

A possible criticism of specific therapy acting solely on production of DHT is that it does not prevent the peripheral conversion of testosterone to oestrogen carried out by the enzyme aromatase. Oestrogen may be important in addition to DHT in the genesis of BPH, by an action predominantly on the stromal component of the prostate. The only aromatase inhibitor which has so far been investigated in clinical studies (testolactone) is a relatively weak antagonist; it has been investigated in an uncontrolled fashion but was found to improve symptoms in 7/13 patients [68], and in half of the treated patients it decreased prostatic size by 15% − 26% [61]. This is an area which warrants further investigation.

Adrenergic Blockade

Learmonth [45] reported that stimulation of the pre-sacral nerve in man contracts the prostatic musculature. Total neural blockage using spinal anaesthesia produces a 47% reduction in urethral closure pressure [26], and α-blockade similarly results in a decrease in urethral closure pressure [23]. Dynamic changes such as these have in recent years highlighted the potential clinical importance of pharmacological blockade of the motor sympathetic adrenergic nerve supply to the prostate. The degree of magnitude of this may vary rapidly according to the level of sympathetic stimulation acting on the prostate gland [26].

Benign prostatic enlargement of the prostate comprises both hypertrophy and in particular hyperplasia of prostatic stromal and glandular compartments. Indeed, contrary to popular belief morphometric quantification of this tissue has suggested that hyperplasia of the stromal compartment is the predominant feature [6]. Although these authors did not carry out a separate analysis of the smooth muscle, it is likely that this would demonstrate a relative increase in the muscular component as contrasted to normal prostate.

Laboratory Studies

The results of in vitro pharmacological isometric studies demonstrate that there is a functional predominance of α_1-adrenoceptors in human prostatic muscle. Radioligand studies demonstrate an overall predominance of $\alpha_1:\alpha_2$-receptors of approximately $3:1$, which is in accordance with the results of the functional studies [15, 40]. A potential source of error exists if there are significant differences in innervation and histological structure between different areas of the same gland. We have carefully investigated this possibility by examining tissue from a number of different areas within prostatic adenomata removed at the time of open operation, and although there was significant regional variation, this appeared to occur randomly with no clearly identifiable regional trends. From these observations it can be concluded that the principal motor control of the prostate is via an action on α_1-adrenoceptors, which are localised predominantly within the stromal compartment of the prostate. These results provide a scientific basis for the use of α_1-adrenoceptor antagonists in the provision of symptomatic relief to selected patients with BPH.

Clinical Studies

The initial clinical application of adrenergic blockade to the lower urinary tract utilised the combined α_1- and α_2-adrenergic antagonist phenoxybenzamine, producing encouraging improvements in urinary flow and clinical symptoms in most clinical studies [1a, 2, 7, 11, 12, 31], with few exceptions [8]. The incidence of side effects in 30% of patients on treatment with phenoxybenzamine [12], combined with evidence of mutagenicity in baterial and mouse cell cultures [4], has despite its clearly documented efficacy precluded its more widespread acceptance in the treatment of benign prostatic obstruction. These adverse effects have been attributed to the blockade of pre-synaptic α_2-adrenoceptors, which is thought to interfere with the normal negative feedback control of noradrenaline release at the pre-synaptic adrenergic nerve terminal, resulting in high circulating nonadrenaline levels.

With recognition of the importance of the α_1-receptor in mediating sympathetic action in the normal and adenomatous prostate, attention has turned to the therapeutic use of selective α_1-antagonists such as prazosin [63], with the intention of reducing unwanted side effects. Prazosin was introduced as an anti-hypertensive agent in 1977 [13] and was subsequently reported to produce urinary incontinence [66, 67]. This incidental observation contributed to recognition of the potential

Table 4. Studies on the efficacy of alpha-adrenoceptor antagonists in improving urinary flow rate

Reference	Treatment period (weeks)		Mean increase in maximum flow rate (ml/s)		Mean increase in mean flow rate (ml/s)	
	n		ml/s	%	ml/s	%
Phenoxybenzamine						
Caine et al. (1978) [12]	50	2	6.2	88	3.2	82
Abrams et al. (1982) [2]	41	4	3.1	43	–	–
Brooks et al. (1983) [3]	28	4	0.9	14	–	–
Prazosin						
Hedlund et al. (1983) [34]	20	4	2.0	41	1.1	42
Martorana et al. (1984) [50]	18	2	6.9	96	2.2	48
Kirby et al. (1987) [44]	55	4	4.8	59	–	–
Hedlund and Andersson (1988) [35]	8	4	2.0	28	1.1	29
Chapple et al. (1990) [16]	58	12	3.2	34	–	–
Le Duc et al. (1990) [46]	39	4	5.35	54	–	–
Alfuzosin						
Ramsay et al. (1985) [59]	31	12	0	–	–	
Jardin et al. (1991) [41]	518	26	1.4	11.5	0.9	14
Indoramin						
Iacovou and Dunn (1987) [38]	30	8	10	118	–	–
Chow et al. (1990) [21]	139	8	4.9	59	–	–
Stott and Abrams (1991) [65]	40	4	2.6	39	–	–
Terazosin						
Fabricius et al. (1990) [25]	57	24	4.2	54	2.7	55
Lepor et al. (1990) [47]	39	8	3.6	42	1.9	48
YM 12617 & 617						
Kawabe and Niijima (1987) [42]	77	2	3.0	43	2.3	85
Kawabe et al. (1990) [43]	270	4	3.6	35	2.0	41

role of selective α_1-adrenoceptor blockade as therapy in the lower urinary tract.

The majority of the existing short-term studies have demonstrated that selective α_1-adrenergic blockade can be effective with few adverse side effects. All of the contemporary α-blockers appear to be very similar in terms of pharmacological and clinical efficacy and safety, producing approximately a 50% increase in urinary flow rate with a significant improvement in patients' symptoms (Tables 4, 5). They are a useful addition to the therapy of patients on a waiting list for surgery, where it is contraindicated for medical reasons and for those who not want surgery. Nevertheless, it must be remembered that optimal pharmalog-

Table 5. Studies on the efficacy of prazosin and indoramin in producing symptomatic improvement

Reference	n	Treatment period (weeks)	Obstructive symptoms	Irritative symptoms	Combined symptoms
Phenoxybenzamine					
Caine et al. (1978) [12]	50	2	–	–	Y
Abrams et al. (1982) [2]	41	4	–	–	Y
Brooks et al. (1983) [3]	28	4	–	–	N
Prazosin					
Hedlund et al. (1983) [34]	20	4	Y	N	Y
Martorana et al. (1984) [50]	18	2	–	–	Y
Kirby et al. (1987) [44]	55	4	Y	Y	Y
Hedlund and Andersson (1988) [35]	8	4	–	–	–
Chapple et al. (1990) [16]	58	12	N	N	Y
Le Duc et al. (1990) [46]	39	4	–	N	Y
Alfuzosin					
Ramsay et al. (1985) [59]	31	12	–	Y	–
Jardin et al. (1991) [41]	518	26	Y	Y	Y
Indoramin					
Iacovou and Dunn (1987) [38]	30	8	N	N	Y
Chow et al. (1990) [21]	139	8	–	–	Y
Stott and Abrams (1991) [65]	40	4	N	Y	N
Terazosin					
Fabricius et al. (1990) [25]	57	24	Y	Y	Y
Lepor et al. (1990) [47]	39	8	Y	Y	Y
YM 12617 & 617					
Kawabe and Niijima (1987) [42]	77	2	Y	Y	Y
Kawabe et al. (1990) [43]	270	4	Y	Y	Y

N: No change as compared to placebo; Y: significantly improved as compared to placebo.

ical blockade of α-receptors by producing a relaxation of prostatic smooth muscle is unlikely to produce more than 50% of that to be expected from a surgical prostatectomy [26, 47, 55].

Criticism has been levelled at the current literature which reports the efficacy of selective α_1-blockade, since it is based on detailed study of short treatment periods [69], with little effect on urodynamic parameters other than the urinary flow rate. Certainly, it must be borne in mind that the symptomatic consequences of secondary detrusor instability are the commonest cause of referral to the urologist, and it is possible that longer periods of treatment are required to demonstrate a therapeutic effect.

A report of the results of the first double-blind long-term study reporting the use of prazosin confirmed the observations of prior workers that there is an increase in the mean maximum urinary flow rate (MFR) on treatment. In addition, it provided the first evidence for a significant change in cystometric parameters, with a 19% reduction in maximum micturition pressure [16, 19]. Separate analysis of urodynamic data from stable and unstable sub-groups revealed interesting differences which did not, however, reach statistical significance, possibly owing to the small number of patients in the stable subpopulation (see Fig. 2). Although the MFR was not increased on active treatment in the unstable patients, there was a corresponding 24% reduction in maximum micturition pressure. Conversely, in the stable group, maximum micturition pressure was virtually unchanged, while there was a 53% increase in MFR. The maximum filling detrusor pressure was decreased by 13% on active treatment in the unstable population as compared to an 18% increase in the stable patients. Possibilities include an indirect consequence of a reduction in α-resistance produced by a direct action on prostatic α_1-receptors or a direct effect on the α receptors within the detrusor [56]; these results do provide some support for the latter suggestion. At present it must be concluded that the mechanism of the reduction in voiding detrusor pressure remains unknown, and further experimental work is required to clarify the situation.

The other published long-term studies report the use of the selective α_1-antagonist terazosin [25, 47], indoramin [21, 38], doxazosin [17] and alfuzosin [41, 59]. Some studies used only limited urodynamic evaluation. Indeed, in the study reported by Jardin et al. [41] only 45% of the patients had had a urinary flow rate estimation and only 36% a post-voiding urinary residual prior to entry into the trial. The work reported by Ramsay et al. was the only one which failed to demonstrate any improvement in the urodynamic parameters of outflow obstruction. The other studies all demonstrated a significant increase in urinary flow rate which then decreased on continuing therapy by 1.3 ml/s (29.5%; [47]), 0.6 ml/s (14,4%; [25]) and 1.8 ml/s (67%; [41]), over a subsequent follow-up period at a least 13 weeks. In a subsequent open study of the

→

Fig. 2. Results of a double-blind, parallel-group, 3-month study contrasting prazosin with placebo. In particular, note changes from baseline values of urodynamic variables in the subgroup of patients with stable **(a)** and unstable **(b)** detrusor function in the prazosin and placebo groups. (From [16])

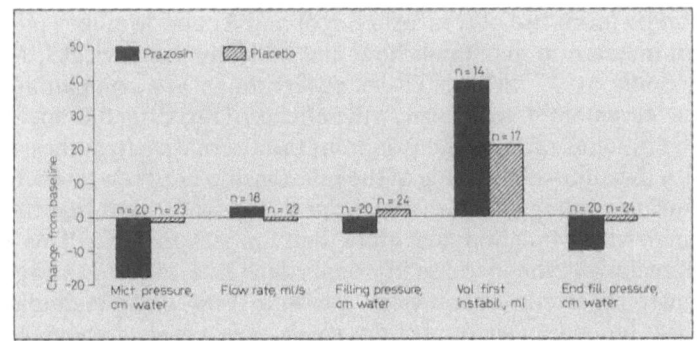

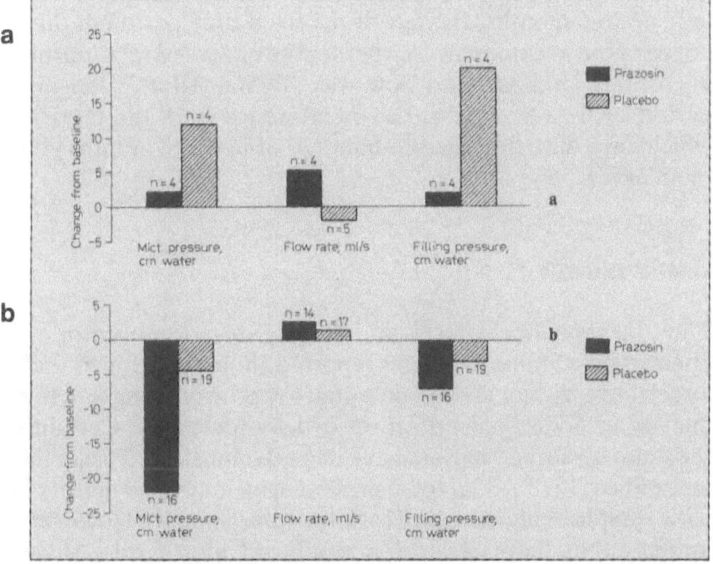

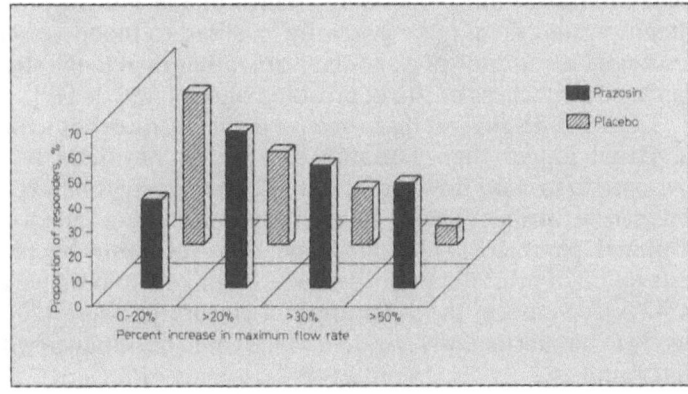

longer terms use of terazosin Lepor and Knapp-Maloney [48] reported an increase in maximum flow rate of 4.7 ml/s at 6 weeks, reducing to 1.6 ml/s at 72 weeks. These observations are compatible with the development of tolerance to the effects of this drug therapy. However, the findings reported here support the alternative hypothesis that there is a dynamic rebalancing of the relationship between pressure and flow during voiding which results from α_1-blockade, and that these effects on detrusor function take more than 1 month to occur. This would also explain why the increase in urinary flow rate was not as large as previously reported in a previous 1-month study using a similar protocol [44]. Indeed, in support of this suggestion it is well recognised that the reduction in detrusor instability which occurs after prostatectomy may take up to 6 months. In view of the fixed time period of this study it is not possible to comment on whether the observed relationship between micturition pressure and flow was maintained at a longer follow-up period such as 6 months, but by inference from the terazosin studies which have data (not double-blinded) of up to 18 months [48] this does seem likely.

Conclusions

The therapeutic effect of the $\alpha_1 - \alpha_2$-adrenoceptor antagonist phenoxybenzamine has been reported to be superior to that achieved by selective α_1-blockade, a potential hypothesis being that this might be due to an additional action on α_2-adrenoceptors. Certainly, human prostatic α_2-adrenoceptors have been demonstrated using ligand binding studies [15, 33, 35a] to be present in an increased density in patients with symptomatic benign prostatic enlargement. However, it seems unlikely that they subserve a significant motor role, since selective slide-mounted autoradiography studies of the human prostate have demonstrated them to be primarily localised to blood vessels and the basement membrane of glandular acini rather than to the stromal compartment, which is the site of prostatic smooth muscle [40].

These results suggest that selective α_1-blockade needs to be given for a period longer than 1 month to achieve maximum benefit. The increase in urinary flow rate is not as great as might be expected, and this can be attributed partly to a reduction in voiding detrusor pressure. Optimal pharmacological blockade of α-receptors by producing a relaxation of prostatic smooth muscle is unlikely to produce more than a 47% decrease in the total urethral closure pressure [26], which is likely to be substantially less than which could be obtained with surgical intervention.

The Future

Laboratory Studies

Laboratory studies need to be directed at the search for more prostate-specific α_1-receptor subtypes, which would allow the development of therapy producing fewer systemic side effects. Selective α_1-blockade of prostatic adrenoceptors using the current non-specific α_1-antagonists is restricted by the systemic (predominantly cardiovascular) side effects which limit the maximum therapeutic dose. Recent animal studies have demonstrated the presence of the α_1-adrenoceptor sub-types, α_{1A} and α_{1B} [53, 58].

We have recently investigated the α_1-adrenoceptor sub-types within the human inferior epigastric artery and prostate [18]. Our preliminary findings suggest that the α_{1B}-adrenoceptor sub-type forms the major population in the prostate, and that α_{1A}-adrenoceptors are predominant in the inferior epigastric artery. Existing α_1-adrenoceptor antagonists have been developed on the basis of their efficacy in the cardiovascular system. Provided that the differences in α_1-receptor subtypes noted between prostate and inferior epigastric artery are repeated on study of other blood vessels in the systemic vasculature. The development of α_{1B}-specific antagonists could improve the therapeutic efficacy of these agents by relaxing prostatic smooth muscle with reduced systemic side effects.

Clinical Studies

Further clinical studies should utilise both comprehensive urodynamic assessment and the detailed analysis of changes in symptoms and investigate the comparability of these two methods of assessing drug efficacy. Work needs to be directed at the investigation of drug combinations, for example, at the potential therapeutic efficacy of the concurrent use of selective α_1-adrenergic blockade to relax the stromal prostatic smooth muscle combined with prostate selective hormonal blockade (e.g., 5α-reductase inhibitors) to shrink the epithelium containing glandular tissue. Additional attention should be directed at parameters which could be used to identify the specific sub-groups of patients likely to respond to pharmacotherapy.

References

1. Abrams PH (1977) A double-blind trial of the effects of candicidin on patients with benign prostatic hypertrophy. Br J Urol 49:67−71
1a. Abrams PH, Shah PJR, Stone AR, Choa RG (1981) Bladder outflow obstruction treated with phenoxybenzamine. Prog Clin Biol Res 78:269−275
2. Abrams PH, Shah PJR, Stone AR, Choa RG (1982) Bladder outflow obstruction treated with phenoxybenzamine. Br J Urol 54:527−530
3. Abrams PH (1985) Detrusor instability and bladder outlet obstruction. Neurourol Urodynam 4:317−328
4. Anonymous (1983) Phenoxybenzamine for symptoms of bladder neck obstruction. Drugs Ther Bull 21:15−16
5. Ball AJ, Feneley RCL, Abrams PH (1981) The natural history of untreated prostatism. Br J Urol 53:613−616
6. Bartsch G, Muller HR, Oberholzer M, Rohr HP (1979) Light microscopic stereological analysis of the normal human prostate and of benign prostatic hyperplasia. J Urol 122:487
6a. Birkoff JD, Weiderhorn AR, Hamilington ML, Zinssen HH (1976) Natural history of benign prostatic and acute urinary retention. Urology 7:48−52
7. Boreham PF, Braithwaite P, Milewski P, Pearson H (1977) Alpha-adrenergic blockers in prostatism. Br J Surg 4:756−757
8. Brooks ME, Sidi AA, Hanani Y, Braf ZF (1983) Ineffectiveness of phenoxybenzamine in treatment of benign prostatic hypertrophy. A controlled study. Urology 21:474−478
9. Cabot AT (1896) The question of castration for enlarged prostate. Ann Surg 24:265−309
10. Caine M, Perlberg S, Gordon R (1975) The treatment of benign prostatic hypertrophy with flutamide (SCH 13521): a placebo-controlled study. J Urol 114:564
11. Caine M, Pfau A, Perlberg S (1976) The use of alpha adrenoceptor blockers in benign prostatic obstruction. Br J Urol 48:255−263
12. Caine M, Perlberg S, Meretyk S (1978) A placebo-controlled double-blind study of the effect of phenoxybenzamine in benign prostatic obstruction. Br J Urol 50:551−554
13. Cambridge D, Davey MJ, Massingham R (1977) Prazosin, a selective antagonist of post-synaptic alpha-adrenoceptors. Br J Pharmacol 59:514P−515P
14. Castro JE, Griffiths HJL, Edwards DE (1971) A double-blind, controlled, clinical trial of spirinolactone for benign prostatic hyperplasia. Br J Surg 58:485−489
15. Chapple CR, Aubry ML, James S et al. (1989) Characterisation of human prostatic adrenoceptors using pharmacology receptor binding and localisation. Br J Urol 63:487−496
16. Chapple CR, Christmas TJ, Milroy EJG (1990) A twelve-week placebo-controlled study of prazosin in the treatment of prostatic obstruction. Urol Int 45 [Suppl 1]:47−55
17. Chapple CR, Carter P, Christmas TJ, Noble JG, Miller P, Kirby RS, Abrams P, Milroy EJG (1991) A three month double-blind placebo controlled study of doxazosin as treatment for benign prostatic bladder outflow obstruction. Neurourol Urodynam 10:308−309
18. Chapple CR, Burt R, Marshall I (1991) α_1 Adrenoceptor subtypes in the human prostate and inferior epigastric artery. Neurourol Urodynam 10:306−308
19. Chapple CR, Stott M, Abrams PH, Christmas TJ, Milroy EJG (1992) A twelve-week placebo-controlled study of prazosin in the treatment of prostatic obstruction due to benign prostatic hyperplasia. Br J Urol (in press)

20. Chisholm GD (1989) Benign prostatic hyperplasia: the best treatment. Br Med J 299:215–216
21. Chow W, Hahn D, Sandhu D, Slaney P, Henshaw R, Das G, Wells P (1990) Multicentre controlled trial of indoramin in the symptomatic relief of benign prostatic hypertrophy. Br J Urol 65:36–38
21a. Clarke R (1937) The prostate and the endocrines: a control series. Br J Urol 9:254–271
22. Craigen AA, Hickling JB, Saunders CRG, Carpenter RG (1969) Natural history of prostatic obstruction. J R Coll Gen Pract 18:226–232
22a. Damrau F (1962) Benign prostatic hypertrophy: amino acid therapy for symptomatic relief. J Am Geriatr Soc 10:426–430
23. Donker PJ, Ivanovici F, Noach EL (1972) Analyses of the urethral pressure profile by means of electromyography and the administration of drugs. Br J Urol 44:180–193
24. Donkervoort T, Zinner NR, Sterling AM, Donker PJ, Van Ness J, Ritter RC (1975) Megesterol acetate in treatment of benign prostatic hyperplasia. Urology 6:580
25. Fabricius PG, Weizert P, Dunzendorfer U, MacHannaford J, Maurath C (1990) Efficacy of once-a-day terazosin in benign prostatic hyperplasia: a randomised placebo controlled clinical trial. Prostate Suppl 3:85–93
26. Furuya S, Kumamoto Y, Yokoyama E, Tsukamoto T, Izumi T, Abiko Y (1982) Alpha-adrenergic activity and urethral pressure profilometry in prostatic zone in benign prostatic hypertrophy. J Urol 128:836–839
27. Garraway WM, Collins GN, Lee RJ (1991) High prevalence of benign prostatic hypertrophy in the community. Lancet 338:469–471
28. Geller J, Bora R, Roberts T et al. (1965) Treatment of benign prostatic hypertrophy with hydroxyprogesterone caproate: effect on clinical symptoms, morphology and of endocrine function. JAMA 193:121
29. Geller J, Nelson CG, Albert JD, Pratl C (1979) Effect of megesterol acetate on uroflow rates in patients with benign prostatic hypertrophy: double-blind study. Urology 14:467
30. Geller (1989) Pathogenesis and medical treatment of benign prostatic hyperplasia. Prostate Suppl 2:95–104
31. Gerstenberg T, Blaabjerg J, Nielsen ML, Clausen S (1980) Phenoxybenzamine reduces bladder outlet obstruction in benign prostatic hyperplasia. A urodynamic investigation. Invest Urol 18:29–31
32. Glynn RJ, Campion EW, Bouchard GR, Silbert JE (1985) The development of benign prostatic hyperplasia among volunteers in the normative aging study. Am J Epidemiol 121:78–82
33. Gup D, Shapiro E, Baumann M et al. (1990) Autonomic receptors in human prostate adenomas. J Urol 143:179–185
34. Hedlund H, Andersson KE, Ek A (1983) Effects of prazosin in patients with benign prostatic obstruction. J Urol 130:275–278
35. Hedlund H, Andersson KE (1988) Effects of prazosin and carbachol in patients with benign prostatic obstruction. Scand J Urol Nephrol 22:19–22
35a. Hedlund H, Andersson KE, Larsson B (1985) Alpha-adrenoreceptors and muscarinic receptors in the isolated human prostate. J Urol 134:1291–1298
36. Huggins C, Stevens RA (1940) The effect of castration on benign hypertrophy of the prostate in man. J Urol 43:705–714
37. Hunter J (1786) Observations on the glands situated between the rectum and the bladder called vesiculae seminales. In: Palmer JF (ed) Collected works, vol 4. Longman, London, p 31

38. Iacovou JW, Dunn M (1987) Indoramin — an effective new drug in the management of bladder outflow obstruction. Br J Urol 60:526–528
39. Isaacs JT (1990) Importance of the natural history of benign prostatic hyperplasia in the evaluation of pharmacologic intervention. Prostate Suppl 3:1–7
40. James S, Chapple CR, Phillips MI, Burnstock G (1989) Autoradiographic analysis of alpha-adrenoceptors and muscarinic cholinergic receptors in hyperplastic human prostate. J Urol 142:438–444
41. Jardin A, Bensadoun H, Delauche-Cavallier MC, Attali P (1991) Alfuzosin for treatment of benign prostatic hypertrophy. Lancet 337:1457–1461
42. Kawabe K, Niijima T (1987) Use of an α_1-blocker, YM-12617, in micturition difficulty. Urol Int 42:280–284
43. Kawabe K, Ueno A, Takimoto Y, Aso Y, Kato H (1990) Use of an $_1$-blocker, YM617, in the treatment of benign prostatic hypertrophy. J Urol 144:908–912
44. Kirby RS, Coppinger SWC, Corcoran MO, Chapple CR, Flannagan M, Milroy EJG (1987) Prazosin in the treatment of prostatic obstruction: a placebo-controlled study. Br J Urol 60:136–142
45. Learmonth JR (1931) A contribution to the neurophysiology of the urinary bladder in man. Brain 54:147–176
46. Le Duc A, Cariou G, Baron JC et al. (1990) A multicenter, double-blind, placebo-controlled of the efficacy of prazosin in the treatment of dysuria associated with benign prostatic hypertrophy. Urol Int 45 [Suppl 1]:56–62
46a. Lepor H (1989) Non-operative management of benign prostatic hyperplasia. J Urol 141:1283–1289
47. Lepor H, Knapp-Maloney G, Sunshine H (1990) A dose titration study evaluating terazosin, a selective, once-a-day α_1-blocker for the treatment of symptomatic benign prostatic hyperplasia. J Urol 144:1393–1398
48. Lepor H, Knapp-Maloney G (1991) Outcome assessment of terazosin for benign prostatic hyperplasia (BPH): 18 month follow-up. J Urol 145:263A
49. Levine AC, Kirschenbaum A, Kaplan P, Droller MJ, Gabrilove JL (1989) Serum prostate-antigen levels in patients with benign prostatic hyperplasia treated with leuprolide. Urology 34:10
50. Martorana G, Giberti C, Damonte P et al. (1984) The effect of prazosin in benign prostatic hypertrophy: a placebo-controlled double-blind study. IRCS Med Sci 12:11–12
51. Matzkin H, Chen J, Lewysohn O, Braf Z (1991) Treatment of benign prostatic hypertrophy by a long-acting gonadotropin-releasing analogue: 1-year experience. J Urol 145:309–312
52. Meiraz D, Margolin Y, Lev-Ran A, Lazebnik J (1977) Treatment of benign prostatic hyperplasia with hydroxyprogesterone-caproate: placebo-controlled study. Urology 9:144
53. Minneman KP (1988) α_1 Adrenergic receptor sub-types, inositol phosphates and sources of cell calcium. Pharmacol Rev 40:87–119
54. Moore RA (1944) Benign hypertrophy and carcinoma of the prostate: occurrence and experimental production in animals. Surgery 16:152–167
55. Noble JG, Chapple CR, Milroy EJG (1991) Long term selective α_1 adrenoceptor blockade versus surgery in the treatment of benign prostatic hyperplasia. Neurourol Urodynam 10:296–298
56. Perlberg S, Caine M (1982) Adrenergic response of bladder muscle in prostatic obstruction. Urology 20:524–527
57. Peters CA, Walsh PC (1987) The effect of nafarelin acetate, a luteinizing-hormone-releasing hormone agonist, on benign prostatic hyperplasia. N Engl J Med 317:599

58. Piascik MT, Butler BT, Pruitt TA, Kusiak JW (1990) Agonist interaction with alkylation-sensitive and resistant α_1 adrenoceptor sub-types. J Pharmacol Exp Ther 204:982−991
59. Ramsay JWA, Scott GI, Whitfield HN (1985) A double-blind controlled trial of a new α-1 blocking drug in the treatment of bladder outflow obstruction. Br J Urol 57:657−659
59a. Rango RC, McLeod PJ, Ruedy J, Ogilvie RI (1971) Treatment of benign prostatic hypertrophy with medrogestone. Clin Pharmacol Ther 12:658−665
60. Roos NP, Wennberg JE, Malenka DJ et al. (1989) Mortality and re-operation after open and transurethral resection of the prostate for benign prostatic hyperplasia. N Engl J Med 320:1120−1123
61. Schweikert HU, Tunn UW (1987) Effects of the aromatase inhibitor testolactone on human benign prostatic hyperplasia. Steroids 50:191−199
62. Scott WW, Wade JC (1969) Medical treatment of benign prostatic hyperplasia with cyproterone acetate. J Urol 101:89
63. Shapiro A, Mazouz B, Caine M (1981) The α adrenergic effect of prazosin on the human prostate. Urol Res 9:17−20
64. Stoner E (1991) Phase 111 studies evaluating 5α-reductase inhibitor and proscar. J Urol 145:57A
65. Stott MA, Abrams PH (1991) Indoramin in the treatment of prostatic bladder outflow obstruction. Br J Urol 67:499−501
66. Straughan JL (1978) Urinary incontinence with prazosin. S Afr Med J 53:882
67. Thien T, Delaere KP, Debruyne FM et al. (1978) Urinary incontinence caused by prazosin. Br Med J 1:622−623
68. Tunn UW, Kaivers P, Schweikert HU (1985) Conservative treatment for benign prostatic hyperplasia. In: Bruchovsky N, Chapdeleine A, Newmann F (eds) Regulation of androgen action. Bruckner, Berlin, pp 87−90
69. Wein AJ (1989) Prazosin in the treatment of prostatic obstruction. J Urol 141:693−694
70. White JW (1895) The results of double castration in hypertrophy of the prostate. Ann Surg 22:1−80
71. Zuckerman S (1936) The endocrine control of the prostate. Proc R Soc Med 29:1557−1568

Some Thoughts on the Mitogenesis of Benign Prostatic Hyperplasia

F. K. Habib[1]

Introduction

Studies undertaken on animals as well as on man support the view that androgens are of importance in the development of benign prostatic hyperplasia (BPH). However, the exact mechanism(s) responsible for initiating and/or sustaining the morphological changes associated with this condition are far from clear.

The prostate gland enlarges only in men with a normal testicular function, and castration usually leads to shrinkage of the gland. Nevertheless, the concentration of dihydrotestosterone (DHT), the active metabolite of testosterone, and its receptor in the hypertrophied gland remain unaltered when compared to the concentration measured in normal prostate tissues [20, 26]. The precise role of androgens in the pathogenesis of BPH is therefore uncertain, and they may permit rather than cause growth. Indeed, increasing evidence suggests that other mitogens might also be involved as regulators of prostate growth [5]. Some of these modulators act in synergy with the steroid hormone to ensure the normal development and function of the gland, whilst others bypass the androgens and imprint their own characteristics on the target cell.

Clearly, further understanding of the events surrounding this all too common condition would have direct clinical relevance in suggesting alternative and more effective treatments for patients with BPH. In this preliminary report attention will be focussed on three factors believed to control intracellular events in the prostate. At a time when simply stopping the supply of testicular androgens has no place in managing BPH [9, 19], interest should now be directed towards the mechanism of

---

[1] University Department of Surgery (WGH), Western General Hospital, Crewe Road South, Edinburgh EH4 2XU, UK

growth within the gland; it would be advantageous to reduce the relative size of the prostate without the adverse side effects usually associated with the manipulation of blood steroid hormone levels.

Prolactin

In addition to recording the sensitivity of prostate to exogenous oestrogen or castration, Huggins noted that prostatic atrophy in dog was more marked after castration and hypophysectomy than after castration alone [8]. This was attributed to a pituitary-related factor which was subsequently identified as prolactin. Prolactin has since been shown to act both independently and in synergy with testicular and adrenal androgens [21, 24]. The exact mechanism of prolactin action is not understood, but the action is believed to be mediated in human tissue by membrane receptors [13], and it is apparent that these receptors accentuate the response of the sex organs to androgens.

Evidence supporting this statement includes the following:

1) A significantly higher uptake of radiolabelled testosterone into benign hyperplastic prostates has been demonstrated in patients with artificially elevated plasma prolactin levels than in controls [3].
2) Androgen uptake in the prostate has been shown to be suppressed in patients taking the prolactin suppressant bromocriptine [10].
3) In addition, an association between blood prolactin and androgen receptors has been shown in BPH [17]. Blood prolactin may exert its action by regulating the 5α-reductase activity and the androgen receptor concentration of the prostate, and this could form the basis for further studies in patients with BPH.

Significantly, no longitudinal study of plasma prolactin and its relation to androgen receptors and 5α-reductase activity in the prostate has been reported. The longitudinal study is of considerable importance in view of the wide range of normality for plasma prolactin. In other words, serial samples must be compared with the patient's own baseline value for meaningful results. The correlation with the presence or absence of a 5α-reductase and androgenic receptors within the tissue is also of importance, as only those patients having high prolactin levels and with a high 5α-reductase activity and androgen receptor positive adenomas at diagnosis would be expected to respond to prolactin suppressants. This hypothesis is at present being tested in our laboratory, and hopefully we will be able to report some interesting results in the not too distant future.

Tissue Interactions and Growth Factors

There is now growing evidence that chemical signalling in the form of soluble growth factors is involved in maintaining cell communication and phenotypic expression in the prostate. In support of this hypothesis are the observations of stromal regulation of epithelial differentiation demonstrated during the development of the prostate and of other glandular structures in the foetus [1]. Many studies have since sought to identify and characterise these diffusable factors, and much attention has focussed on those derived from prostatic tissue [12, 23]. Hirata and Orth [7] were the first to demonstrate the presence of epidermal growth factor (EGF) in the human prostate using a radioimmunoassay. Growth factors other than EGF are also associated with this gland. Maehama et al. [15] characterised a growth factor derived from rat ventral prostate. This rat prostate-derived growth factor (rPrDGF) was distinct biologically from other growth factors such as EGF, fibroblast growth factor (FGF), and transforming growth factor (TGFα and TGFβ); however, rPrDGF has some biochemical similarities to TGFβ. Jacobs and Lawson [11] reported on the presence of a second fibroblast growth promoting factor in crude extracts of BPH, well-differentiated carcinoma and postpubertal normal prostate. This growth factor was distinct from EGF and TGFα in that it did not compete for the EGF receptor [23], and it was also distinct from FGF in that the components were acidic and not basic [12]. Additionally, Nishi and coworkers [16] purified a growth factor from cytosol preparations of human benign adenoma which was capable of stimulating DNA synthesis of BALB/3T3 cells; this growth factor differed from bovine FGF and EGF. More recently, nerve growth factor and nerve growth factor receptor biosynthesis in the glandular epithelium in prostate adenomas was also established [2].

Clearly the prostate is a focal point for diverse peptide activities, but whether any of these growth factors are involved in the hyperplastic process remain to be seen. Some recent findings suggest, however, that certain peptides may be involved in the pathogenesis of BPH. Measurement of EGF concentrations in prostate fluid from BPH patients and normal subjects indicate a significantly higher EGF concentration in specimens obtained from subjects with normal prostates and no evidence of outflow obstruction [4]. Differences in secretion may be related to a retention mechanism associated with the development of BPH. Confirmation of this hypothesis stems from the studies on the expression of EGF receptors in prostate tissue: whilst 94% of all BPH specimens exhibit detectable levels of the EGF receptor [14], normal prostate obtained from cadaver organ donors under 30 years of age revealed no or few receptors [6]. This raises the possibility that the up-regulation of EGF receptors in BPH might be related to the development of this condition, but whether as a cause or as a result remains to be elucidated.

The control of prostatic cell proliferation is a complex process involving numerous interactions. Some interactions require cell-to-cell contact [18], whereas others are mediated by externalised cellular matrices or soluble factors [22]. In order to identify the nature of these cell-to-cell interactions which may occur in adult human prostate, and to identify the mechanism that may be involved, attempts should be made to study the effects of combining these separate cell populations of cultured epithelial and fibroblastic cells from human prostate. This will overcome the artefact arising from a non-human model, and the characteristics and growth requirements of prostate epithelial cells derived from normal and hyperplastic tissues could be investigated. The coculture of these cells with fibroblasts derived from the prostate of the same patient will also offer a unique opportunity to study in vitro the stroma/epithelial interactions of an adult human organ system.

Genetic Factors in BPH

The conversion of normal cells to the fully metastatic phenotype is a complex phenomenon resulting from the activation/repression of a number of specific genes. One of the determinants underlying the progress to a tumour is the order of genetic alterations, which follow a cascade of events starting with the normal cell presumably free of acquired mutations and gradually progressing via early, intermediate and late adenoma to a cancer which finally metastasises. Each of these stages is characterised by the gain or loss of a wide variety of gene products.

The concept that BPH is a precursor for cancer of the prostate has been repudiated repeatedly over the years. The bulk of experts are of the opinion that the pathobiologies of the two diseases are unrelated and that induction of BPH follows a pathway totally distinct from that charted by cancer of the prostate (CaP). Even so, no one has yet karyotypically characterised BPH and CaP and reliably classified the chromosomal patterns. Evidence derived from studies of different stages of colorectal neoplasia support our model in which accumulated alterations affecting at least one dominantly acting gene and several tumour suppressor genes are responsible for the development of colorectal tumours [25]. The progressive nature of these genetic alterations initially promotes the transition from hyperproliferative epithelium to the adenomatous state, and one cannot at this stage ignore the possibility that a similar process might underlie the development of BPH.

This is an interesting concept which could be tested very rapidly employing the modern advances in molecular biology. Our team in Edinburgh is already proceeding along these lines with very promising results. Although the work is still in its infancy, the results are encouraging, and if they prove consistent this could lead to the use of reverse genetics and antisense technology in the management of benign prostatic hyperplasia.

References

1. Cunha GR, Donjacour AA, Cooke ES, Mee S, Bigsby RM, Huggins SJ, Sugimora Y (1987) The endocrinology and developmental biology of the prostate. Endocrine Rev 8:338−362
2. Dicoue E, Saint-Andree GB, McGrogin D (1991) Nerve growth factor (NGF) and NGF receptor biosynthesis in human prostatic adenomas and in cell lines derived from prostatic carcinomas. Prog Urol [Suppl]1:7
3. Farnsworth WE, Slaunwhite WR, Sharma M, Oseko F, Brown JR, Gonder MJ, Kartagena R (1981) Interaction of prolactin and testosterone in human prostate. Urol Res 9:79−81
4. Gregory H, Wiltshire IR, Kavanagh KP, Blacklock NJ, Chowdury S, Richards RC (1986) Urogastrone/epidermal growth factor concentration in prostate fluid of normal individuals and patients with benign prostatic hypertrophy. Clin Sci 70:359−363
5. Habib FK (1990) Peptide growth factors: a new frontier in prostate cancer. In: Newling DWW (ed) Prostate cancer and testicular cancer. Liss, New York, pp 107−115 (EORTC Genito-Urinary Group monograph 7)
6. Habib FK, Chisholm GD (1991) The role of growth factors in the human prostate. Scand J Urol Nephrol [Suppl] 126:53−58
7. Hirata Y, Orth DN (1979) Epidermal growth factor (urogastrone) in human fluids: size, heterogeneity. J Clin Endocrinol Metab 48:673−679
8. Huggins C, Russells PS (1946) Quantitative effects of hypophysectomy on testes and prostate of dogs. Endocrinology 39:1−7
9. Huggins C, Stevens RA (1940) The effect of castration of benign hypertrophy of the prostate in man. J Urol 43:705−714
10. Jacobi GH, Sinterhauf K, Kurth KH, Altwein JE (1978) Bromocriptine and prostatic carcinoma: plasma kinetic production tissue uptake and radiolabelled testosterone in vivo. J Urol 119:240−243
11. Jacobs SC, Lawson RK (1988) Mitogenic factors in human prostate extracts. Urol 16:488−493
12. Jinno H, Ueda K, Otazuro K, Kato T, Ito J (1986) Prostate growth factor and extracts of benign prostatic hyperplasia. Eur Urol 12:41−48
13. Leake A, Chisholm GD, Habib FK (1983) Characterisation of the prolactin receptor in human prostate. J Endocrinol 99:321−328
14. Maddy SQ, Chisholm GD, Hawkins RA, Habib FK (1987) Localization of epidermal growth factor receptors in the human prostate by biochemical and immunocytochemical methods. J Endocrinol 112:147−153
15. Maehama S, Saline D, Nanri S, Leykm JF, Deuel TF (1986) Purification and characterisation of prostate derived growth factor. Proc Nat Acad Sci USA 83:8162−8166

16. Nishi M, Matuo Y, Mugurama Y, Yoshitake Y, Nishikawa K, Wada F (1985) Human prostatic growth factor (hPGF): partial purification and characterisation. Biochem Biophys Res Commun 132:1103−1109
17. Odoma S, Chisholm GD, Nicol K, Habib FK (1985) Evidence for the association between blood prolactin and androgen receptors in BPH. J Urol 133:717−720
18. Ohkawa H, Harigay K (1987) The effect of direct cell to cell interaction between the KM-102 clonal human marrow stromal cell line and the HL-60 myeloleukaemic cell line on the differentiation and proliferation of HL-60 line. Cancer Res 47:2879−2882
19. Peters CA, Walsh PC (1987) The effect of nafarelin acetate, a lute inising hormone releasing hormone agonist, on benign prostatic hyperplasia. New Engl J Med 317:599−604
20. Robel P, Eychanne B, Blondeau JP, Baulieu EE, Hechter O (1985) Sex steroid receptors in normal and hyperplastic human prostate. Prostate 6:255−267
21. Slaunwhite WR, Sharma M (1977) The effect of hypophysectomy and prolactin replacement therapy on prostatic response to androgen orchiectomised rats. Biol Reprod 17:489−492
22. Sporn MB, Todaro JG (1980) Autocrine secretion and malignant transformation of cells. New Engl J Med 303:878−880
23. Story MD, Jacobs SC, Lawson RK (1983) Epidermal growth factor is not the major growth promoting agent in extracts of prostatic tissue. J Urol 130:175−179
24. Thomson SA, Heidger PM (1978) Synergistic effects of prolactin and testosterone in the restoration of rat prostatic epithelium following castration. Anat Rec 191:31−45
25. Vogelstein B, Fearon ER, Hamilton SR et al. (1988) Genetic alterations during colorectal tumour development. New Engl J Med 319:525−532
26. Walsh PC, Hutchins GM, Ewing LL (1983) Tissue content of dihydrotestosterone in human prostatic hyperplasia is not super normal. J Clin Invest 72:1772−1777

Endocrinology of Normal and Pathological Development of the Prostate

P. Bonnet and C. Bouffioux[1]

Introduction

The prostate as much as other accessory sexual glands (e.g., seminal vesicles, bulbourethral glands) has been used for a long time as a model for the study of the mechanism of action of androgens on the regulation of protidic and ribonucleic synthesis toward understanding regulation of the secretory activity and epithelial growth. The prostate is present in mammals only. It produces various components of the spermatic fluid, including fructose, zinc ions, and protides. In human pathology, benign prostatic hypertrophy (BPH) is the most frequent non-malignant proliferative disease.

Histologically, BPH can be found in fewer than 10% of men under the age of 30 years. The incidence increases with age and reaches 50% in the fifth decade and 80% in the eighth decade [1, 25]. The risk for a man aged 40 years for developing BPH requiring surgical treatment is approximately 10% [7, 17]. The etiology of BPH remains mysterious but endocrinological factors − mainly involving androgens − seem to play a part. For this reason, various hormonal treatments − medical or sometimes surgical − have been proposed as an alternative to the classical surgical management of BPH. We review here the hormonal pathways responsible for the development of prostatic gland and the facts suggesting their participation in the genesis of BPH.

[1] Centre Hospitalier Universitaire, Service d' Urologie, Domaine Universitaire du Sart Tilman B 35, B-4000 Liege I, Belgium

Hormonal Pathways

Hypothalamo-Hypophysis Axis and Peripheral Targets

The hypophysis secretes various peptidic hormones under hypothalamic control; these include luteinizing hormone (LH), follicle-stimulating hormone (FSH), growth hormone (GH), adrenocorticotropic hormone (ACTH), prolactin (PRL), and thyroid-stimulating hormone (TSH). Gonadotropin-releasing hormone (GnRH) is released by a pulse secretion from the hypothalamus and reaches the anterior pituitary through the pituitary portal system. This basal pulsatile secretion (once per hour) does not require suprahypothalamic stimulation and is modulated by several neurotransmitters, such as norepinephrine, dopamine, histamine, and endorphine. Testosterone, aromatized locally in estradiol, and estradiol itself produce a negative feedback which regulates GnRH secretion. Gonadotropic cells of the anterior pituitary stimulated by GnRH secrete LH and FSH. LH enters the blood circulation; it has a half-life of 50 min (6 h for FSH). FSH stimulates spermatogenesis and the secretion of low levels of estrogens by Sertoli's cells. Inhibin produces a negative feedback on the pituitary. LH stimulates the steroidogenesis of Leydig's cells. Estrogens and testosterone cause a negative feedback. The negative feedback of testosterone is more potent for the secretion of LH than for that of FSH.

The testis, stimulated by LH, secretes testosterone, the major circulatory androgen in men. Ninety-eight percent of plasma testosterone is bound to transport proteins: sex hormone binding globulin (SHBG; high affinity), albumin (low affinity but large capacity), and other proteins that are less important such as transcortin, progesterone-binding globulin, and alpha-acid glycoprotein. Only 2% of plasma testosterone is free and able to react with target organs. In the peripheral tissues, testosterone (a steroid hormone) diffuses through the cellular membrane. In some cells (in the muscles, testis, or vas deferens) testosterone reacts directly with the cytosol receptor. However, in the hairy follicles or the epithelial cells of the prostate, testosterone is first converted into Dihydro testosterone (DHT) by the enzyme 5-alpha-reductase. DHT has a much higher affinity than testosterone for androgen receptors. The complex androgen receptor is translocated into the nucleus where derepression and transcription of genes occur with synthesis of messenger RNA and finally synthesis of peptides responsible for the final action of androgens on the cell, including differentiation, secretion, and growth.

PRL is secreted by the anterior pituitary under hypothalamic control, whether stimulating (thyrotropin-releasing hormone) or inhibiting (prolactin-inhibiting factor, dopamine). PRL acts on the mammary gland, modulates the testicular steroidogenesis, and seems to have an action on the prostatic cells directly or by modulation of the androgenic effects. Under hypothalamic control the pituitary also secretes TSH, ACTH, and GH, which influence the growth and metabolism of many tissues. The role of these hormones in the prostatic diseases is not prominent [23].

Other Endocrine, Paracrine, and Autocrine Influences

The prostatic cells are also, like all the other cells, under the influence of autocrine and paracrine factors (insulin, insulin-like growth factor, epidermal growth factor, etc.). Many growth factors are currently being studied, but it is still too early to define their role in the development and pathology of the prostate gland or to predict the value of their antagonists in the treatment of BPH [19, 29].

Endocrinology of the Development of the Prostate

Many observations have established the crucial role of androgens in the embryological growth of the prostate. The removal of the testes or medical castration during the ambisexual period inhibits the development of the male sexual glands, including the prostate [15, 24]. In organ culture, testosterone is able to induce the formation of prostatic structures even from a female urogenital sinus [3, 16, 22, 26]. During the postnatal period, the development of the prostate remains under the control of androgens; castration prohibits the development of the gland, which may be restored by addition of testosterone [2, 21]. In the cases of natural deficiency in 5-alpha-reductase or in the presence of inhibitors of this enzyme, the prostate gland remains rudimentary [11–13]. Genotypic males without androgen receptors (testicular feminization, TFm) display a female phenotype with a complete absence of prostatic tissue [9, 20, 27, 28].

Hormonal Regulation of Adult Prostate

Prostatic morphology and activity is androgen dependent. In humans and animals, medical or surgical castration causes regression of the prostate as indicated by a decrease in DNA synthesis, decrease in the weight of the gland, and regression of the epithelial component more important than that of the stroma. If exogenous androgens are given, one observes a restoration of the gland. Other hormones also play a role in the adult prostate. Receptors for estrogens, progesterone, and PRL have been identified, but their role is less important. In dog BPH, estrogens seem to act synergically with androgens [6].

Role of the Different Components of the Prostatic Gland: Epithelium and Stroma

Intrinsic factors seem also to play a role in the development and the functional integrity and activity of the prostate. Experiments performed by Cunha and coworkers have shown the interrelation between the epithelial and the stromal tissue. If glandular tissue from an adult male rat prostate is grafted under the kidney capsule of another adult male rat, it survives but does not grow. If embryonic or neonatal prostatic tissue is grafted in the same conditions, one observes the development of a complete prostate. This difference in the behavior of the graft may be explained by the inductive role of the stromal tissue on the gandular component. In the embryonic and neonatal prostates, the stroma is predominant while the epithelial tissue is the most important in the adult prostate. Other experiments by Cunha have clearly shown the inductive role of the prostate mesenchyma on the epithelium, even on an epithelium of different origin and insensitive to androgens [4, 5].

Is BPH a Disease due to Hormonal Disturbances?

BPH develops in two stages [14]. There is a microscopic stage where micronodular organization appears as early as age 25−30 years. The incidence increases with age and reaches 100% at age 85−90. The disease remains subclinical. A macronodular stage is due to the growth of the micronodules, starting around age 35−40 years. Its incidence is about 50% in men aged 80 years. MacNeal's studies have clearly demonstrated that these nodules appear in two precise areas of the prostate: the periurethral zone, where the nodules are mainly stromal, resembling the embryonal mesenchyma, and the transitional zone, where growths is mainly glandular [18]. The etiology of BPH remains controversial, but some considerations seem to indicate that hormones, in particular androgens, play some role in the occurrence of the disease: (a) true eunuchoids and men castrated before puberty have no BPH, and (b) after castration or hormonal manipulation there is some evidence of regression of the disease [14].

Is There a Specific Hormonal Environment
Favoring the Development of BPH?

Studies performed in this area are confronted with major difficulties. First, there is no adequate animal model. Indeed, only man and dogs naturally develop BPH. In dogs this hypertrophy is only epithelial, in contrast to man in whom the fibromuscular stroma plays an important part. Secondly, BPH arises in several stages, starting at age 25–30 years and progressing to the end of life. For this reason, longitudinal studies are impossible. The study of BPH at a precise time offers only a short view of a pathology initiated many years earlier. Thirdly, the universality of the disease, at least in its micronodular stage, does not allow controls with disease-free populations in the same age groups.

Various studies have tried to define, sometimes contradictorally, the hormonal environment accompanying BPH, an environment which, in fact, corresponds to that of the aging man. Total plasma testosterone remains unchanged or decreases slighthly through the sixth or seventh decade of life, with subsequent progressive reduction thereafter. There is no consensus concerning differences in circulating testosterone levels in „normal" age-matched men and BPH patients. Similarly, the relationship between total plasma DHT and BPH in elderly men remains unclear. SHBG increases in aging men, and this increase could be more important in BPH patients. These proteins enter the prostatic cells, and this could explain the accumulation of SHBG-like proteins observed in BPH tissue. Estrogens are produced mainly by peripheral aromatization of androgens in the fatty tissue. Testes aromatize 10%–25% of estradiol. These estrogens are linked to SHBG and to albumin; only 2% remains free in the plasma. The principal estrogen-dependent morphological responses in male accessory sex organs are squamous epithelial metaplasia and fibromuscular stromal growth. Estrogens influence androgen uptake and metabolism in the human prostate. In addition, estrogens indirectly influence levels of free steroids in the plasma and their uptake into accessory sex organs by stimulating increases in SHBG levels. The estrogen/androgen ratio in aged men is elevated compared to values found in younger age groups. This finding apparently results from increased estrogen and unchanged or decreased androgen levels in the elderly. Estrogens may be important in the etiology of BPH, considering the observations of an increased estrogen/androgen ratio with age, the possible synergism of estrogens with androgens in epithelium, and the estrogenic stimulation of prostatic fibromuscular stromal growth.

Whereas adrenal androgens may be important in castrated men, their possible role in the etiology of BPH in aged men appears negligible. An age-dependent increase in circulating gonadotropins occurs in men, although the increase is not of the large magnitude as observed in postmenopausal women. This increase in gonadotropins in men has been presumed to result from disinhibition of the negative feedback mechanism secondary to an age-dependent decrease in testicular function. There are no apparent BPH-related alterations in FSH levels, but there is no consensus regarding differences in levels of circulating LH in BPH patients versus those in age-matched controls. In vitro growth rates of human BPH have also demonstrated a synergistic action of PRL on androgen action. Although basal PRL levels have been demonstrated in some studies to be increased in BPH patients compared to those in controls, other laboratories were unable to demonstrate significant differences.

Are There Hormonal Changes Within the Gland Explaining the Outcome of BPH?

DHT 5-Alpha-Reductase. DHT (the result of reduction of testosterone by cytoplasmic 5-alpha-reductase) has for a long time been considered an important factor in the development of BPH. Some studies have indicated an accumulation of DHT in BPH, but further investigation showed, that this accumulation was partly due to technical problems and early tissular alterations occurring in the prostates of cadavers. Nevertheless, 5-alpha-reductase activity is increased in preparations of fresh BPH tissue. 5-Alpha-reductase should be concentrated mainly in the stroma of normal or hypertrophic prostate. Two different isoenzymes were identified with different characteristics for the stroma and for the epithelium. The increased activity of 5-alpha-reductase in BPH compared to normal prostate is considered by some investigators as a sign of a tissue endocrinologic change producing a hormonal etiology of the disease.

Estrogens, FSH, LHRH, and Other Hormones. Receptors for estrogens, progesterone, and luteinizing hormone releasing hormone are found in BPH tissue. Their role in the pathophysiology of BPH, if any, is not well established.

Epithelium Stroma Interactions. The particular organization of BPH nodules looks like the embryologic prostatic tissue organization, where the importance of epithelium-stroma interactions is clearly demonstrated. Thus some investigators think that BPH may be due in part to the activation of embryologic properties in a special hormonal environment [8, 10].

Conclusions

The development and function of the prostate undoubedly depend upon hormonal influences, among which the hypothalamic-hypophysis axis plays a predominant role. BPH is a consequence of a slow process requiring, at least in its initial phase, a normal androgenic environment. The interactions between the epithelium and the stroma and the emergence of embryonal capacities probably also play an important role in this disease. There is a little evidence that hormonal treatments given at an advanced stage of a disease developing over several decades will produce a complete regression of the affection. One can expect only a limited efficacy.

References

1. Berry SJ, Coffey DS, Walsh PC, Ewing LL (1984) The development of human benign prostatic hyperplasia with age. J Urol 132:474–479
2. Berry SJ, Isaacs JT (1984) Comparative aspects of prostatic growth and androgen metabolism with aging in the rat versus the dog. Endocrinology 114:511
3. Cunha GR (1973) The role of androgens in the epithelio-mesenchymal interactions involved in prostatic morphogenesis in embryonic mice. Anat Rec 175:87
4. Cunha GR, Chung LWK, Shannon JM, Reese BA (1980) Stromal-epithelial interactions in sex differentiation. Biol Reprod 22:19
5. Cunha GR, Donjacour AM (1987) In: Coffey DS, Chiarodo A, Karr JP (eds) Currents concepts and approaches to the study of prostate cancer. Liss, New York, pp 251–272
6. Cunha GR, Donjacour AM, Cooke PS, Mee S, Bigsby RM, Higgins SJ, Sugihuma Y (1984) The endocrinology and developmental biology of the prostate. Endocr Rev 8/3:338–362
7. Ekman P (1989) BPH epidemiology and risk factors. Prostate Suppl 2:23–31
8. Geller J (1989) Pathogenesis and medical treatment of benign prostatic hyperplasia. Prostate Suppl 2:95–104
9. Griffin JE, Wilson JD (1984) Disorders of androgen receptor function. Ann NY Acad Sci 438:61
10. Hinman F (1984) Section III endocrine control. In: Hinman F (ed) Benign prostatic hypertrophy. Springer, Berlin Heidelberg New York, pp 175–313
11. Imperato J, McGinley J (1984) 5α-Reductase deficiency in man. Prog Cancer Res Ther 31:491
12. Imperator J, McGinley J, Guerrero L, Gautier T, Peterson RE (1974) Steroid 5α-reductase deficiency in man: an inherited form of pseudohermaphroditism. Science 186:1213
13. Imperato J, McGinley J, Peterson RE, Gautier T (1984) Primary and secondary 5α-reductase deficiency. In: Serio M, Zanisi M, Martini L (eds) Sexual differentiation: basic and clinical aspects. Raven, New York, p 233
14. Isaacs JT, Coffey DS (1989) Etiology and disease process of benign prostatic hyperplasia. Prostate Suppl 2:33–50
15. Jost A (1953) Problems of fetal endocrinology: the gonadal and hypophyseal hormones. Rcent Prog Horm Res 8:379

16. Lasnitziki I, Mizuro T (1977) Induction of rat prostate gland by androgens in organ culture. J Endocrinol 110:467
17. Lyhon B, Emery JM, Haward BM (1967) The incidence of benign prostatic hypertrophy. Trans Am Assoc Genitourin Surg 59:65—71
18. McNeal JE (1985) Morphology and biology of benign prostatic hyperplasia. In: Bruchovsky N, Chapdelaine A, Neumann F (eds) Regulation of androgen action. Proceedings of an international symposium, Montreal 1984. Brückner, Berlin, pp 23—30
19. Nishi N, Matuo Y, Kunitomi K, Takenaka I, Usami M, Kotake T, Wada F (1988) Comparative analysis of growth factors in normal and pathological human prostates. Prostate 13:39—48
20. Ohno S (1979) Major sex determining genes. Springer, Berlin Heidelberg New York, p 1
21. Price D (1936) Normal development of the prostate and seminal vesicles of the rat with a study of experimental postnatal modifications. Am J Anat 60:79
22. Price D, Ortiz E (1965) The role of fetal androgens in sex differentiation in mammals. In: DeHaan RL, Ursprung H (eds) Organogenesis. Holt, Rinehart and Winston, New York, p 62
23. Rajfer J (1986) Chapters 6 and 7. In: Rajfer J (ed) Urologic endocrinology. Saunders, Philadelphia
24. Raynaud A, Frilley M (1947) Destruction du cerveau des embryons de souris au treizième jour de la gestation, par irradiation au moyen des rayons X. C R Soc Biol (Paris) 141:658
25. Schröder F, Blom JHM (1989) Natural history of benign prostatic hyperplasia (BPH). Prostate Suppl 2:17—22
26. Takeda I, Lasnitzki I, Mizuno T (1986) Analysis of prostatic bud induction by brief androgen treatment in the fetal rat urogenital sinus. J Endocrinol 110:467
27. Wilson JD, Griffin JE, George FW, Leshin M (1984) Recent studies on the endocrine control of male phenotypic development. In: Serio M, Zanisi M, Martini L (eds) Sexual differentiation: basic and clinical aspects. Raven, New York, p 223
28. Wilson JD, Griffin JE, Leshin M, George FW (1981) Role of gonadal hormones in development of sexual phenotypes. Hum Genet 58:78
29. Wilson EM, Smith EP (1987) Growth factors in the prostate. In: Coffey DS, Chiarodo A, Karr JP (eds) Current concepts and approaches to the study of prostate cancer. Liss, New York, pp 205—233

New Forms of Hormonal Treatment in Benign Prostatic Hyperplasia: Efficacy of Flutamide

H. W. Bauer[1]

During the past 20 years there has been renewed interest in the hormonal treatment of benign prostatic hyperplasia (BPH) based on the development of new pharmacological agents and the general desire of patients to avoid an operation. As long as the hormonal treatment of BPH is based on the idea of malfuncting endocrine regulation of the prostate, it seems reasonable to block the ailing system at various metabolic levels. While effects on BPH remain the same regardless of the level (metabolic passway) blocked, striking differences in sexual function result.

Effective antiandrogenic agents are flutamide and cyproterone acetate. Antiandrogenes interfere with the binding site of androgen receptors or the translocation of the androgen receptor complex in the nucleus. Cyproterone acetate has additional progestational and antitrogenic activity which causes sexual impotence.

The first results came from Scott and Wade [1]. They treated 13 patients with cyproterone acetate and achieved subjective improvement in 11. Maximum urinary flow rate was increased while volume of residual urine decreased in 9 and 8 patients, respectively. This nonrandomised, non-placebo-controlled study showed for the first time that symptomatic BPH can be treated effectively with pharmacological methods designed to inhibit growth of the prostate. The impact of this study was limited owing to the small number of patients examined and the failure to evaluate clinical efficacy critically.

A second study on antiandrogenic drugs in BPH was conducted by Caine and coworkers [2]. This was the first double-blind placebo-controlled study design in the treatment of BPH. A total of 30 patients with symptomatic BPH received 100 mg flutamide 3 times per day for 12 weeks. Urinary flow rates improved significantly and relief of subjective symptoms was noted. Principal adverse effects were gynecomastia

---

[1] Maximilianstraße 31, W-8000 München 22, FRG

and tenderness of the nipples in 7 patients of the verum group while libido and sexual potency were preserved. Both studies were carried out before the availability of routine ultrasound measurement of prostate volume and residual urine and failed to differentiate between obstructive and irritative symptoms. With sonographic measurements it has become possible to reevaluate antiandrogenic therapy with this method.

A pilot study was conducted by Bauer et al. [3]. Included were 30 patients (27 available) with a sonographic prostate volume of more than $60 cm^3$. Intraindividual changes in residual and subjective symptoms were accounted. Final results were compared to those gathered in the 3-month pretreatment period. The patients received 3 × 250 mg flutamide per day for 16 weeks. All patients benefitted from the treatment in terms of subjective symptoms; no aggravation was seen. A significant reduction of residual urine volume was achieved in 11/27 patients. No change was seen in 10 patients while in 6/27 an increase in residual urine volume was observed. Sonographically measured prostatic volume was reduced by more than 30% in 9/27 patients. The coefficient of variation for multiple measurements was 10%. While sexual function was unchanged (maintained) in all patients, adverse effects such as gynecomastia and pain in the nipples were reported in 10/27 (Table 1).

To determine a dose-related effect of flutamide on both the prostate and the mammarian gland a two-armed study over 12 weeks with 3 × 250 mg flutamide (group A) versus 2 × 250 mg flutamide (group B) was conducted. There were 80 patients with BPH-induced bladder outlet obstruction included in this prospective randomized two-armed multicenter study [4] (Table 1). In both groups there was a subjective

Table 1. Results with flutamide in antiandrogenic hormonal therapy of BPH

	Bauer et al. [3]	Bauer et al. [4]
Subjective improvement	14/27	A: 33/41 B: 33/41
Residual urine	11/27 reduction >25% 10/27 no change 6/27 increase	A: 36/41 reduction >20% B: 31/41 reduction >20%
Prostatic volume	9/27 reduction >30%	A: 15/32 reduction >30% B: 6/28 reduction >30%
Libido, sexual potency	No changes	Diminished in 2 patients
Adverse reactions: pain in the nipple, gynecomastia	10/27	A: 17/41 B: 9/41

improvement in 33 of 41 patients. Residual urine was reduced more than 20% in 36/41 of group A and in 31/41 of group B. Prostate volume reduction of more than 30% was seen in 15/31 of group A and in 6/28 of group B.

The most recent antiandrogenic study in BPH therapy is the study conducted by Stone [5]. This was a multicenter, randomized, double-blind, placebo-controlled study with 84 patients. To date patients have reached 12 weeks some even 24 weeks. At 24 weeks a 41% average decrease in prostate volume was seen. In the placebo group no statistical change in prostate volume was observed at 3 or 6 months. Uroflow also did not change in patients receiving placebo but increased by 30% at 12 weeks and 35% at 24 weeks in the flutamide group. There were no severe side affects in the placebo group but in the flutamide group there were four patients (11%) with breast pain, gynecomastia, and diarrhea. Breast pain was experienced in a mild form by 53%; one patient discontinued the treatment because of these symptoms. No patient complained of impotence or change in libido while taking flutamide.

Summary

Antiandrogenic therapy with flutamide is an effective treatment for BPH-induced obstructive symptoms (such as reduced flow rates and residual urine). Preselection of patients who might benefit from this treatment remains a problem. Adverse effects on the mammary gland will hamper general acceptance of this treatment.

References

1. Scott WW, Wade JC (1969) Medical treatment of benign nodular prostate hyperplasia with cyproterone acetate. J Urol 101:81
2. Caine M, Perlberg S, Gordon R (1975) The treatment of benign prostatic hypertrophy with flutamide: a placebo-controlled study. J Urol 114:564
3. Bauer HW, Kühne P, Dieckmann KP, Jonas D (1986) Efficacy of flutamide therapy in human benign prostate hyperplasia. J Urol 135:369
4. Bauer HW, Bach D, Dunzendorfer U, Pensel P (1989) Konservative Therapie der benignen Prostatahyperplasie (BPH) mit Flutamid. TW Urol Nephrol 1:259−269
5. Stone NN (1989) Flutamide in treatment of benign prostatic hypertrophy. Urology [Suppl]34:64−68

The Need for Objective Evaluation of Therapy in Benign Prostatic Hyperplasia

R. A. Janknegt[1]

Introduction

Until recently benign prostatic hyperplasia was treated exclusively by operation, open prostatectomy or transurethral prostatectomy (TURP). Although the indication for the operation was based mainly on subjective criteria such as the complaints of the patients and rectal examination, the results were generally good. The operative success rate as determined by the patient was 85%. Complaints of frequency and nocturia disappeared in most of the patients. Recent publications, however, mention that the overall late outcome following TURP is not as favorable as assumed, and there are suggestions that in cases with minor symptoms prostatectomy may offer far fewer advantages over watchful waiting than previously thought. Approximately 425 000 prostatectomies were performed for BPH in the United States in 1990. Although this comprises a high percentage of the health care costs in the United States, it is amazing that this important operation has very seldom been evaluated by objective criteria (flow, pressure-flow).

With the recent development of new alternative treatment forms such as medication, hyperthermia, dilatation, and spirals there is a need for objective comparison of the various modalities. We discuss here objective and subjective parameters which can be used to evaluate the efficacy of these treatment forms. Comparison can be made only if clear criteria are instituted. New treatment modalities may be compared not only with placebo but also with the natural history of the condition, and comparison can be made with TURP. Although some studies have been made with high quality, most of them contain deficiencies of design, conduct, analysis, or presentation of results. Recently, medical studies have been performed, however, comparing medication with placebo over a long period of time (2 years). Such a

[1] Academic Hospital Maastricht, Department of Urology, P. Debyelaan 25, NL-6202 AZ Maastricht, The Netherlands

study also gives statisticians some idea as to how many patients may be needed if the difference between the medication and the placebo is relatively small.

Ideally, evaluation is based on objective data. Subjective data (symptoms) are generally difficult to quantify and analyze. If new treatment forms with different etiologic concepts, such as reduction in prostate size or dimishing α-adrenergic contractility, are introduced, knowledge of the various types of hyperplasia, such as fibromuscular and adenomatous pathophysiologic changes must be accurately staged, either by ultrasound, computed tomography (CT), or magnetic resonance imaging (MRI). In this context we discuss the use and value of the following parameters: (a) symptom-score, (b) prostate size, (c) flowmetry, (d) residual urine, (e) cystoscopy, and (f) pressure-flow studies.

Symptom Scores

Although symptom scores may be important, because they show the benefit for the patient, they are not quantitative for the effect on the obstruction of the prostate by any new treatment form. Subjective data are generally difficult to quantify and analyze. It is well known that symptom scores may improve without changing the obstruction of the prostate (for example, with placebo). Therefore the symptom score needs statistically significant differences if such scores can be used appropriately. Obviously there is a lack of objective criteria here.

Symptom scores do not take into consideration the effects of the given condition and symptoms on the patient's activities of daily living or quality of life. It is possible to influence the status change that prompted the patient to seek treatment. It is also possible favorably to influence the symptom responsible for the status change without significantly effecting an overall symptom score. An adequate protocol must include a methode for validation of the symptom score. When using symptom scores, comparability of the scores in various studies is necessary. At the moment there are at least three symptom scorescales available: Boyarski et al. [2], Madsen and Iversen [5]. Also the WHO and ICS are at the moment developing new symptom scores.

Although most of these use a seven-point question system, the difference between obstructive and irritative symptoms is not the same. Obstructive symptoms occur during the emptying phase and include hesitancy, decreased stream, a feeling of incomplete emptying, straining to void, and intermittency of stream. These symptoms are characteristic of bladder outlet obstruction or impaired detrusor contractility.

Irritative symptoms occur during the filling phase of the bladder and generally include daytime frequency, urgency (urgent incontinence), and nocturia. These are associated with involuntary bladder contractions.

A comparison of the symptoms in a group of elderly men without prostatism and an age-matched group of patients showed marginal differences. One may conclude that abnormalities from the normal are quite often interpreted differently.

Irritative symptoms may be the result of outlet obstruction leading to instability of the bladder. Abrams [1] found detrusor instability in 53%−80% of all patients with outlet obstruction. Release of the obstruction may reverse this phenomenon. A decrease therefore in irritative as well as obstructed symptoms may be due to a release of obstruction. However, urgency may also occur from a bladder that empties very poorly and is in overflow. Symptom quantification and interpretation is difficult.

Prostate Size

Prostate size is not important for the degree of obstruction. If the three lobes provide a sufficient gutter, even large lobes may not lead to obstruction. However, small prostates with a high amount of contractile fibromuscular components may lead to severe obstruction.

Prostate size can be measured directly, by ultrasound, or by MRI. Rectal examination assesses only part of the prostate (posterior and lateral portions). Even with the same examiner, consistent ratings may differ. Evaluation therefore is highly subjective, and when comparing sizes with an in-between period of 1−2 months, the reproducibility varies from examiner to examiner. Ultrasonography is probably the best and most reliably available reproducible form of total prostate size estimation. Measuring prostate weight after radical prostatectomy showed a good correlation with ultrasound. CT and MRI are obviously accurate methods, but expensive and time consuming. They can be used only for specific studies with a small number of patients. Ultrasound holds the promise of being able to detect different metabolic or size changes and perhaps differences in epithelial from stromal forms. When studying the use of 5α-reductase or other hormonal treatments which diminish the size of the prostate, an objective and good parameter, such as accurate ultrasonography, must be used.

Flowmetry

Although diminished flow may be caused by either outlet obstruction or impairment of detrusor contractility, it is acknowledged that most men with bladder outlet obstruction have a diminished flow rate and altered flow pattern. When using flowmetry as a parameter, the definition of pathology versus normal in the various age groups, should be clearly stated. There are computer programs available which may be of help in analyzing pathology versus normal. Siroky et al. [4, 5] developed nomograms for average and maximum flow rates based on flow rate measurements in a group of younger men. Flow rates, however, depend upon initial bladder volume. They found relatively small variability in a single individual's flow rate over time and concluded that urinary flow rate, when statistically related to initial bladder volume, could be used to estimate outflow resistance. It is presumed that a urine flow lower than 10 ml/s shows obstruction, and that a flow rate of more than 15 ml/s excludes obstruction. However, this does not take into consideration the age of the patient. A recently published set of maximum and average urine flow rates in normal male and female populations (Liverpool nomograms), agreed that a certain amount of deterioration in male urinary flow rates occurs with age. It is doubtful that consistency will be achieved among flow nomogram makers. However, this is one of the systems that may be utilized for comparison following treatment of BPH.

Residual Urine

If residual urine is present, its reduction in volume is an important parameter in the evaluation of results of treatment of BPH. However, as patients come earlier with their complains, most patients with BPH nowadays have a minimal residual urine volume.

In most patients with a significant residual urine it is impossible to differentiate deficient bladder contractility from outlet obstruction as the primary etiology without a pressure-flow study. Catheter measurement of the residual volume obviously is the most accurate means, but it is invasive, causes discomfort, and may introduce infection. Noninvasive methods include isotope scanning and sonography. However, these are more expensive and usually less accurate. Also, it is very unfortunate that most patients have a wide variation of residual urine volumes at different times.

Cystoscopy

Cystoscopy does not contribute to objective evaluation of either obstruction or detrusor contractility. It is used for identifying other causes of obstruction (strictures, bladder neck sclerosis) or irritability (bladder stones or tumors).

Pressure-Flow Studies

Flow can be defined as the relationship between obstruction and detrusor contractility. Outlet obstruction is characterized by a poor flow rate in the presence of a detrusor contraction of adequate force and duration. When there is obstruction, the detrusor pressure generally rises, and the flow rates generally fall. Also the flow rate shape becomes more plateaulike and parabolalike.

Obstruction causes detrusor changes such as muscle hypertrophy and trabeculation. The reaction of the bladder muscle is divided into three phases: irritation, compensation and decompensation. Therefore it is essential to differentiate the state of the bladder muscle. Cystometry gives a good answer to the situation of the detrusor. However, simultaneous measurement of bladder pressure and flow may be jeopardized by a transurethral catheter. Therefore, cystometric measurements should be done by suprapubic catheters.

Recent developments in the area of cystometry have lead to new objective parameters which make it possible to differentiate between obstruction and decreased detrusor contractility. Software computer programs such as CLIM may help in the measurement of these parameters. Several studies have now shown that patients with evident prostatism complaints are classified as unobstructive in 25% of all patients. Whether such measurements are necessary to evaluate the response of BPH to the various treatment forms, or how much they add to the evaluation of the efficiency of a drug or procedure is as yet unsettled. Several nomograms have been developed to understand the relationship of obstruction versus detrusor contraction (Schaefer nomogram, Van Mastrigt CLIM program). Although these invasive studies may be the most accurate in urodynamically describing response of treatment, they should be the last performed to complete the profile of action of a given drug or procedure on BPH.

Another consideration which should be kept in mind is the dissociation between symptoms and urodynamic improvement, which occurs with the same treatment form. It is not yet clear whether this dissociation between symptomatic improvement and mild or nonimprovement urodynamically indicates that there is some ill-defined mechanism within the prostatic urethra that is not directly related to the amount of mechanical obstruction.

Discussion

We now know that BPH is a heterogeneous disease combining dynamic factors (α-adrenergic overstimulation, cholinergic understimulation) and static factors (variations in size by adenomatous versus fibromuscular hyperplasia). The various treatment forms have different targets aiming at correction of any of these factors. Efficacy must be measured by comparison. In medication studies it is possible to perform placebo studies. However, with hyperthermia placebo studies are more difficult. Comparison with the gold standard (TURP) so far is not possible in most studies.

Not only the improvement of flow, question score and pressure flow should be kept in mind but also the late results of treatment forms; short-term and long-term effects may be quite different in the various treatment arms.

Future studies should consider: (a) pathologic status of the prostate (adenomatous versus fibromuscular tissue); (b) symptom score versus quality of life; (c) pressure-flow studies in phase I and phase II studies (but are not essential for all patients); (d) long-term follow-up as the final goal (1–10 years); and (e) costs factors (a life-long medication versus a single operation). Studies should be double blind and randomized for all new treatment forms. Before evaluating any of the new treatment forms for BPH there must be a better definition of the result, including objective parameters such as pressure-flow measurements. Treatment forms should also state the late goals such as long-term effects. Technology assessment of the various forms is eminently necessary.

Conclusion

When assessing the efficacy of new alternative treatment forms, strict objective criteria should be used. Symptom scores and flowmetry give indications of patient improvement and changes in either obstruction or bladder contractility. Urodynamic assessment by pressure-flow studies are the only available methods that allow objective differentiation of obstruction or impaired detrusor contractility and are reproducible. As 25% of all patients with prostatism are unobstructed, pressure-flow studies must be included in the evaluation of efficacy of new treatment forms for BPH.

References

1. Abrams PH (1985) Detrusor instability and bladder outlet obstruction. Neurol Urodynam 4:317
2. Boyarsky S, Jones G, Paulson DF, Prout GR (1977) A new look at bladder neck obstruction by the food and drug administration: guidelines for investigation of benign prostatic hypertrophy. Trans Am Assoc Genitourin Surg 68:29−32
3. Brich NC, Hurst G, Doyle PT (1988) Serial residual volumes in men with prostatic hypertrophy. Br J Urol 62:571
4. Haylen BT, Sahby D, Sutherst JR et al. (1989) Maximum and average urine flow rates in normal male and female populations − the Liverpool nomograms. Br J Urol 64:30
5. Madsen PO, Iversen P (1983) A point system for selecting operative candidates. In: Hinman F Jr (ed) Benign prostatic hypertrophy. Springer, Berlin Heidelberg New York, pp 763−765
6. Peters CA, Walsh PC (1987) The effect of naferelin acetate, a lutinizing hormone releasing hormone agonist on benign prostatic hyperplasia. N Engl Med 317:599
7. Rollema HJ, Van Mastrigt R (1991) Objective analysis of prostatism: a clinical application of the computer program CLIM. Neurourol Urodynam 10:71−76
8. Schafer W, Rubben H, Noppeney R et al. (1989) Obstructed and unobstructed prostatic obstruction: a plea for urodynamic objectivation of bladder outflow obstruction in benign prostatic hyperplasia. World J Urol 6:198
9. Siroky MB, Olsson CA, Krane RJ (1979) The flow rate nomogram: I. Development. J Urol 122:665
10. Siroky MB, Olsson CA, Krane RJ (1980) The flow rate nomogram: II. Clinical correlations. J Urol 123:208

Transurethrale Microwave Thermotherapy (TUMT) in Patients with Benign Prostatic Hyperplasia (BPH)*

R. Laduc[1]

Symptomatic BPH is normally treated with a transurethral or open prostatectomy. These operations are effective and relatively safe. Mortalit is less than 1 percent [1].

There is, however, a considerable morbidity, both directly after the operation and later. Urethral strictures are found in 2−22% [2−4].

Re-resection is necessary in 2−16% of the operated patients [3]. Other complications are urinary retention, clot retention, urinary tract infection and incontinence. The frequency of erectile dysfunction after prostatectomy is not well established. Although it is not a complication, retrograde ejaculation is present in over 50% of the operated patients. The resulting infertility can be a problem, especially in younger males. Other disadvantages of prostatic surgery are the need for general or regional anaestesia and hospital admission.

In recent years several alternative treatments for BPH have been proposed. Drugs as phenoxybenzamin and prazosin are known to be effective. They diminish the infravesical obstruction by relaxation of the smooth muscle cells in the prostate and the bladder neck (α-adrenergic blocking agents). In a therapeutic dose half of the patients have serious side effects like dizzines, low blood pressure and visual disturbances. A volume reduction of the prostate with 20% or more can be obtained with hormonal treatment. Flutamide has probably no negative effect on potency [5], but has the disadvantage of side effects also. Recently, the effects of finasteride were tested on a large scale, both in the USA and Europe. Some improvement in peak flow and also a moderate improvement in the severity of the symptoms were shown. A new drug, atamestan, is presently tested in several centres in Europe.

---

* The unusual position of this manuscript in the book is due to the delay.
[1] Akademisch Ziekenhuis Nijmegen, Urologie, Geert Grooteplein 16, NL-6500 HB Nijmegen, The Netherlands

Results of balloon dilatation of the prostate are not clear [6]. Prostate stenting has to be seen as an alternative for a transurethral catheter.

In this article we would like to focus on hyperthermy and thermotherapy.

Heating the prostatic tissue can be done transrectally or tgransurethrally. Irreversible damage of normal tissue can be obtained if temperatures are reached of 45°C or more [7]. After a healing proces of this damaged tissue, shrinkage of the prostate can be expected [8].

If we want to reach these temperatures in a considerable part of the prostate, even higher temperatures are needed near the antenna. This because of the loss of heat energy by absorption of the tissue and by the cooling effect of the circulating blood. As a consequence, tissue necrosis will be the result near the antenna. If a transurethral route is chosen, bleeding and pain will be the effect. More seriuous is the possibility of necrosis of the rectal wall with transrectal application of heat energy. To prevent these risks, many of the available machines will give only limited amounts of energy with a temperature of less than 45°C near the energy source. Intraprostatic temperatures are even lower. To be effective it is advocated to repeat treatment sessions up to 10 times.

In our clinic we have used the Prostatron machine (Technomed) since October 1990. With the Prostatron we are able to reach thermotherapeutic temperatures in the prostate. Treatment consists of one single outpatient session of 60 minutes duration. A transurethral catheter is inserted and positioned with the aid of transabdominal ultrasound. The microwave antenna reaches temperatures well above 45°C (up to 55 to 60°C) deep into the prostatic tissue. Necrosis of the urethral mucosa is prevented by a cooling system incorporated in the catheter. The circulating fluid keeps the temperature below 44.5°C near the catheter, while deeper in the prostatic tissue still high temperatures can be reached because of the radiative heating. Urethral and rectal temperatures are constantly measured to prevent necrosis while giving energy up to 60 Watts.

Since October 1990 more than 300 patients were treated with this method in our department. Inclusion criteria for TUMT treatment were a peak flow of less than 15 cc/sec on two occasions with a prostate volume of at least 30 cc. Main exclusion criteria were an isolated enlargement of the middle lobe of the prostate, a residual urine of more than 250 cc, suspicion of a carcinoma of the prostate, and other causes of prostatism complaints as urethral strictures or neurogenic bladder fucntion disturbances.

A minority of the patients (18%) needed anti-pain treatment during the procedure. Only in 1.5% treatment had to be stopped for this reason. Introduction of the catheter failed in another 1.5%. Technical problems were encountered in the first months of using this machine, preventing or interrupting the treatment in another 6% of the patients. Due to edema of the prostatic tissue, urinary retention developed in 26% of the patients. A transurethral catheter was given for a period of 5 to 7 days. In all patients the catheter could be removed succesfully. Bleeding after the procedure was only slight and of short duration. 3 patients had bleeding for a longer period, on cystoscopic examination, this was seen to be caused by damage of the mucosa. In one patient, blood was seen coming from the seminal vesicle.

Treatment results are now evaluated. In general, some improvement of uroflowmetric parameters was seen. There was a clear reduction of symptoms (more than 50% reduction in Madsen symptom score) after 6 weeks, which was still present after 3 and after 6 months. PSA values raised from an average of 4.6ng/ml to 24ng/ml after two weeks. 6 weeks after treatment PSA was normal again. Semenanalysis is 10 patients before and 3 months after treatment showed no change. No retrograde ejaculation was seen. At present, no statistically significant reduction of the prostate volume could be shown.

Conclusion

Several non operative treatment modalities for BPH patients are developed. If they will be a good alternative for prostatectomy is not sure. A longer follow up period is necessary in hyperthermy and thermotherapy. Also, studies comparing TUR-P and TUMT will have to be undertaken.

References

1. Kristensen MM, Bruskewitz RC (1990) Clinical manifestations of BPH and indication for therapeutic intervention. Urol Cl N (amer) 17:509
2. Mebust WK (1990) Transurethral Prostatectomy, Urol Cl N (amer) 17:575
3. Bruskewitz RK et al. (1986) Three year follow up of urinary symptoms after TUR-P. J Urol, 136:613
4. Nielsen KK, Nordling J (1990) Urethral strictures following TUR-P, Urology, 36:18
5. Stone NN (1989) Flutamide in the threatment of BPH, Urology (suppl.) 34:64
6. Reddy PK et al. (1990) Balloon dilatation of the prostate for treatment of BPH. Urol Cl N Amer, 17:529
7. Harzmann R, Weckermann D (1991) Lokale Hyperthermie bei Prostataerkrankungen?, Akt Urol, 22:10
8. Devonec M et al. (1991) Transurethral Microwave Heating of the prostate, J Endourol, 5:129